CHART II

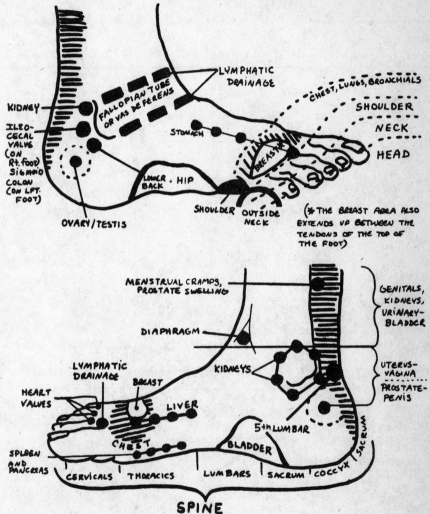

KIDNEY

ILEO-CECAL VALVE (ON RT. FOOT) SIGMOID COLON (ON LFT. FOOT)

FALLOPIAN TUBE OR VAS DEFERENS

LYMPHATIC DRAINAGE

STOMACH

LOWER + HIP BACK

OVARY/TESTIS

SHOULDER OUTSIDE NECK

BREAST

CHEST, LUNGS, BRONCHIALS

SHOULDER

NECK

HEAD

(*THE BREAST AREA ALSO EXTENDS UP BETWEEN THE TENDONS OF THE TOP OF THE FOOT)

MENSTRUAL CRAMPS, PROSTATE SWELLING

DIAPHRAGM

LYMPHATIC DRAINAGE

BREAST

KIDNEYS

HEART VALVES

LIVER

CHEST

5th LUMBAR

BLADDER

SACRUM

GENITALS, KIDNEYS, URINARY-BLADDER

UTERUS-VAGINA

PROSTATE-PENIS

SPLEEN AND PANCREAS

CERVICALS   THORACICS   LUMBARS   SACRUM   COCCYX

SPINE

THE FOOT BOOK

Healing the Body through Foot Reflexology

DEVAKI BERKSON, M.A.

Illustrations by the Author
Photographs by Joseph A. Graffeo

HarperPerennial
A Division of HarperCollins*Publishers*

To everyone's feet, I wish you gentle comfort and love. Tread softly and grow.

My special wish is that we grow to have the kind of feet and feeling that, wherever we've passed, people who later walk that path will feel refreshed and inspired though they know not why.

A hardcover edition of this book was published in 1977 by Funk & Wagnalls. It is here reprinted by arrangement with Funk & Wagnalls.

HarperCollins books may be purchased for educational, business, or sales promotional use. For information, please call or write: Special Markets Department, HarperCollins Publishers, Inc., 10 East 53rd Street, New York, NY 10022. Telephone: (212) 207-7528; Fax: (212) 207-7222.

First Barnes & Noble Books edition published 1979. First HarperPerennial edition published 1992.

LIBRARY OF CONGRESS CATALOG CARD NUMBER 91-58520

ISBN 0-06-092296-6

92 93 94 95 96 C W 10 9 8 7 6 5 4 3

Contents

Introduction

One of the preoccupations in our long lives has been the importance of health.

Hundreds of people have written or visited us asking us to share our general life style, particularly our thoughts and practices on establishing and preserving good health.

As part of the stream of young people passing through our homestead, Devaki Berkson impressed us with her vigor, vitality, resourcefulness, and outgoing determination to make a personal contribution to the health and well-being of the earth and its inhabitants.

Her studies were pointed healthward through her college training. Latterly, as a student of chiropractic, she has been devoting her full attention to health: its nature, its preservation, and its improvement.

In this research about health she has been particularly concerned with the close connection between physical well-being and mental poise.

We are of like mind in this particular and are therefore more than glad to add our good wishes and our hopes that this book will provide encouragement and practical assistance to many a health seeker.

Helen and Scott Nearing

Preface

I had been ill for some time. I had seen doctors and had undergone operations. Yet all this still left me in the midst of misery, bewilderment, and pain, as if I were about to fall off a craggy cliff while no one knew what to do, or cared.

Fate fumbled me into the hands of a foot reflexologist. I began regular treatments. My diet was reformed, and I started a specific exercise program. In a short time my problems lessened, then disappeared without ever returning.

That experience convinced me to study reflexology and health from all levels. Academically I earned a master's degree in nutrition. Physically I studied yoga, massage, polarity, and shiatsu and became a certified shiatsu therapist. For the past several years I have been conducting seminars and retreats in exercise, physiology, nutrition, and massage to share my good fortune with my fellowmen.

Foot reflexology becomes more fascinating, more healing, and more incredible each year and with each treatment.

As long as an action is imbued with a certain moral energy, I honestly believe it doesn't matter what we do in life, but how we do it. Anything we do in the end is but an excuse to confront and solve problems—in other words, to learn how to give to our fellowmen. Reflexology is one of the best gifts God could have shown us to learn how to reach out, touch, and serve His creation.

In reviewing the literature, one discovers occasional differences of opinion regarding techniques and the positions of reflex points. But I have found that if one works the foot thoroughly and sincerely, the results are all positive.

I feel there is no *one* way to give a treatment. There is no need to idolize one method or teacher. Each healer must find his or her own way. However, finding one's own way comes from learning and mastering previous teachings, then "growing up" and going beyond the teachers.

The Integrated Treatment we discuss in this book is not of the past. It is a vital treatment making room for intuition and encouraging new discoveries.

The reflexology programs may be used by the layman. They are not to be thought of as cure-alls. One should not hesitate to contact a licensed physician if necessity or good judgment so dictates.

Devaki

Acknowledgments

I should like to give a big "thank you" to Bill Eastman, without whom this book would never have been possible. Thanks and devotion go to Christ, Swami Satchidananda, Helen and Scott Nearing, and Yogi Bhajan, whose teachings have guided me on this path.

Appreciation goes to my mother, father, and brother (Eleanor, Abraham, and Denis Berkson), Dan McGuire, Troy and Lylas Clark, Chuck Balford and Tricia Knoll, Renée and John Rose, and Jeffery Fitzhum for their support in the production of the manuscript.

A Note to the Reader

You are a human being, a child of the Universe. You have
a right to feel good. And you have the ability to be a channel
for healing and an aid to those around you.

You can help yourself. You can help others. You can help
by learning and becoming proficient with simple healing
tools. The Integrated Treatment is a very simple, very
powerful healing tool.

One warning: Edgar Cayce once said when someone
asked him to define sin that "Sin is knowledge not lived."
So, if you are about to read this book and learn what it has
to offer, please use it. When you are first learning, do at
least one foot massage a day so it sticks with you. Don't be
a book faddist who reads, collects, and talks a lot, but then
stands by doing nothing when a friend is in need. If someone has a headache and you see him reach for an aspirin, or
just complain, give that person a foot treatment. Touch
him. Reach out. Practice and become fuller and fuller by
giving more and more. Give yourself up to giving. Know
that by giving a treatment you are also receiving one.

Reflexology and the Art of Healing

Simply stated, reflexology is an ancient therapy designed to bring the body back into healthful balance after it has lost its center due to wrong living, illness, and pain, and to provide preventive maintenance, which is a daily must.

Reflexology is based on the premise that our organs have corresponding reflex points on other parts of the body, some of the most sensitive points being those on the feet. These corresponding points are found by dividing the body into different zones. Organs lying in a particular zone can be stimulated by pressing various reflexes in the corresponding reflex point zone. All the organs over the entire body have reflex points in the feet. These reflexes appear on the foot charts (I–IV) included as endpapers in this book. These reflexes are five to twenty times more sensitive than the organs themselves. Thus, the foot is a scanner screen recording bodily functions. Tender reflexes are easy to find on the feet, and make it possible to know which organs are not functioning properly. Working tender reflexes helps rebalance these organs. Accordingly, organ maintenance and the lessening and elimination of pain and discomfort can be achieved by applying therapeutic action to those reflex points corresponding to the organs in question.

Good health is a matter of balance. From the organs to these reflex points there are pathways, or currents, through which pass the all-important energy our bodies need to maintain balance and vibrancy. These energy currents can be mapped on the body as highways are marked on a map. Reflexology releases the blocks that don't allow the body's energy currents to flow properly. The methodology is simple, much like learning to push the right buttons (reflex points) on a computer (the body) to balance the energy of the body and allow good health to permeate the entire system. When a reflex point is stimulated, it works to balance and normalize not just the corresponding organ itself but also all functional relationships of that organ. When stimulated, the heart reflex on the bottom of the foot helps balance not just the energy flow of the heart but also the circulation, lymph and venous drainage, and can even assist in normalizing menstruation.

Different schools of healing have varying systems of dividing and labeling the paths of our energy currents. They may be called zones, meridians, electromagnetic currents, and even chi', to name but a few. Neither are they always conceived of as moving in the same direction or on the same areas of the body. But all these systems do deal with the body in terms of flowing energy.

Up to now, no one has been able to explain in precise scientific terms why reflexology works, but recent studies and experience with acupuncture and related therapies are revealing findings that are helpful in bringing a fuller explanation to reflexology.

This book is about feet and the therapy of foot reflexology. Yet it is more than mere foot reflexology; several different schools of healing have made major contributions toward a balanced life, and to omit them would be wrong. So together with foot reflexology we shall combine elements of Swedish massage, polarity, shiatsu, and zone therapy to arrive at an integrated foot treatment. Foot treatment is presented as a coordinated health program that involves diet, exercise, and the use of healing visualizations and affirmations. In this respect you should think of this book as being concerned with the entire system of good health. The broad treatment it espouses we call the "Integrated Treatment."

There really is so much more to good, balanced health than just ridding oneself of pain and discomfort. The Integrated Treatment desires that the body be an example of vigor, of top physical condition, of vibrant energy, and one that sends forth positive vibrations. It offers a well-rounded and balanced system of healing because the maintenance and fulfillment of life should be well rounded and balanced.

Furthermore, it works. And that is what we are interested in—something that works with lasting and gentle results.

I am more and more convinced that diet, exercise, and attitude are each equally important contributors to good health; one is as important as the other. Neither a "perfect diet" nor positive thought, by itself, is a panacea. There is no *one* answer. We must look at the whole story:

> We are what we eat,
> We are what we do, and
> We are what we think!

The Integrated Treatment is inspiring enough, easy enough, and truly effective enough so that, when combined with foot reflexology:

> What we do will be healing,
> What we eat will be strengthening, and
> What we think will be uplifting.

It would be well to spend some time here thinking about the art of healing, for one who practices the Integrated Treatment indeed becomes a healer. And for clarity, throughout the book the person giving the treatment is referred to as the practitioner. The person receiving the treatment is called the patient.

You, the healer and the practitioner of the art, have certain responsibilities which in turn become rewards for you as well as for the person healed.

Developing the art of healing is best approached from two levels: the spiritual and the physical.

On the spiritual you must open yourself up to become a channel for healing energy. This is done through visual imagery, affirmations, and relaxation techniques.

On the physical you must learn the proper techniques and treatment such as diet, massage, and reflexology. You must also train yourself to be a detective by being concerned with the whole person, by taking your time and never jumping to conclusions, and by searching out each symptom as a challenge.

Being a detective is where much of the real art of healing lies, for you must regard the patient carefully:

- Do you judge the skin coloring to be healthy?
- How easily do the joints rotate?
- Which reflex points are the most tender or the most difficult to relieve?
- Is the posture abnormal, as if carrying a heavy burden?
- Is there resistance or tenseness in the muscles?
- Are the heels of the shoes worn evenly?
- Are the eyes and tongue clear or coated?
- What about the nails and hair? Are they strong and shiny, or are they brittle?
- What about the patient's mental attitude when discussing his problem?
- Do you notice a nervous laugh? Is there a twitch?
- Is the skin clammy or blotched?

It's like the old parlor game of "Clue" and finding out who killed Mrs. White in the library with a pipe. These symptoms are all clues that will lead the health detective to the solution of his patient's problems. While we shall be discussing symptoms in greater detail later in the book, it is worth recognizing now that a healer is concerned with the whole person—it is the most perfect wholeness of the patient's being that the healer seeks to restore.

In perfecting the art of healing, there are important practices that will help you greatly:

- Be aware. This involves observing, recording, and testing yourself. Notice as many details about the patient as possible—color of the eyes, the most common facial and body expressions. Memorize them and write them down. Test yourself when the patient is with you and your eyes are closed. Test yourself again when the patient is gone.

- Learn to listen. Observe the speech patterns, the voice tone, the articulation. Be aware of each word and movement. Is the patient really in touch with his problem, or is he fooling himself?
- Learn to touch. Become more comfortable about feeling skin and holding and moving people's feet. Touch as many people as you can in a therapeutic manner. Learn to recognize tension and resistance under your fingertips; learn to recognize relaxation and resilience. Be aware of tone, temperature, and texture.
- Study the foot charts. When you touch real people, relate what you feel to what you see. At the outset keep illustrations and charts at your side when you give treatments.
- Study in general. Improve yourself by attending lectures, classes, and seminars. Read to expose yourself to what is going on in the field and for background information.* Become acquainted and comfortable with basic physiology and anatomy. Acquaint yourself with natural healing and cleansing processes. Understand that sometimes things become worse in the process of becoming better.
- Become healthy yourself. Live what you profess. Recognize the fact that others respond to your healing and advice at the level at which you live it yourself. Being the best healer means focusing healing on yourself. The only thing you can ever teach is what you really are. If you are an example, your life becomes your most powerful teaching.
- Be patient. Pain and disease are seldom gone in a day. Patience also begets confidence within your patients.

The art of healing through the Integrated Treatment recognizes the need for an unobstructed flow of energy throughout the human body, and the universal healing forces that are present throughout the universe at all times. Our Creator and the divine forces of nature do not mean for us to be at the mercy of every disease and negative influence that fate and past actions blow our way. The Integrated Treatment helps prevent illness; it lets the waters of repair and healing flow when disease and negative influences are active.

* Recommended books: 1. McNaught and Callander, *Illustrated Physiology*, Churchill Livingstone, New York, 1975. 2. I. MacKay Murray, M.D., *Human Anatomy Made Simple*, Doubleday & Company, Inc., New York, 1969. 3. Carmine D. Clemente, *Anatomy: A Regional Atlas of the Human Body*, Lea & Febiger, Philadelphia, 1975.

"But," you may ask, "why do we concentrate on the feet? Why not some other part of the body?"

True, there are other places on the body that contain all the reflex points for the entire body. Dr. Ralph Alan Dale has named these "micro-acupuncture systems." In these areas many of the energy pathways of the body converge, and nerve fibers from all the organs are directly or indirectly represented. In fact, all micro-acupuncture systems have a placement of reflex points that echoes the anatomy of the human fetus. The known areas of the body having all the reflex points are the wrist (that is what makes Asian pulse diagnosis possible), the foot, hand, ear, neck, abdomen, face, head, arms and legs, nose, the iris of the eye (this is what makes iris diagnosis possible), and the tongue. So, by treating any one of these areas, the entire body is benefited, not only specifically but also generally.

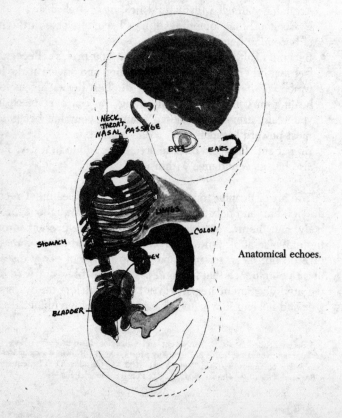

Anatomical echoes.

But the feet are one of the most effective body areas on which to practice reflexology because:

- They are such strong energy poles of the body, and they link with the energy emanations from the earth, especially from the grass, sand, and snow.
- They are one of the most comfortable and non-threatening areas of the body on which to work.
- Due to the constant gravity forces on our feet and to constant wear and tear, they accumulate large deposits of acids and tensions. These affect the health of the entire person.
- Here build-up of acidic crystals (i.e., lactic acid) and hardening from tissue degeneration can readily be felt, seen, and treated.
- Touching the feet is a gesture that soothes and deeply affects a person. For thousands of years a hospitable host washed the feet of his guests. It is impossible to wash feet thoroughly without inadvertently massaging them.
- It is easy to understand from our charts the body's anatomical representation on the feet.
- The reflex points on the feet are more sensitive than any other reflex points. Because feet are frequently covered with shoes and socks, they remain quite tender. Furthermore, there is less musculature between the massaging hands and the reflex points of the feet than there would be on most other parts of the body.
- Finally, feet are a link between the infinite energy of the universe and the finite energy of humans. Jesus washed the feet of His disciples at the Last Supper, thereby linking their lives to His, thus cleansing, protecting, and blessing their whole being.

So, with integrated reflexology we combine diet, exercise, and the use of healing visualizations and affirmations to give us the Integrated Treatment. But we may also consider the Treatment from four points of view: the physical, the mental, the spiritual, and as an art.

- *The Physical.* This affects the organs and circulation by re-establishing, unblocking, and stimulating blood, oxygen, nutritional and energy pathways. Tension is released, nerve activity is balanced, and congestion and other deposits are thrown off. The overall vitality of the body is increased, making true relaxation and activity possible.

- *The Mental.* The act of one person helping another, especially through touch is an effective therapy in itself. Reflexology soothes and calms. This, much more than just a therapeutic situation, becomes an act of giving and receiving—a real sharing of true communication between two people. It also stimulates the body's own personal powers of regeneration and self-repair, leaving positive and lasting emotional results. The resulting feeling of confidence and calm encourages the body to become stronger and better able to service itself.

- *The Spiritual.* On the spiritual plane, too, reflexology is a powerful act of communication between two persons. The practitioner is blessed with the opportunity to serve, and the patient is blessed with the opportunity of receiving healing. Together they call upon the healing forces of the universe to surround, permeate, and uplift. During the treatment, the vibrations, the energy, and the motives of practitioner and patient are closely interrelated and influenced. Service and purity are important to healing; one must rise above the desires of laying negative and sensual emotions on one's partner. The use of affirmations and projecting positive healing is a spiritual act. It is prayer in action. Reflexology, then, is a divine gift whereby we can be of service to others. We all possess healing powers of the universe within us, and we all have the right and ability to call upon the healing power of God, nature, or whatever we feel comfortable calling it.

- *The Art.* The Integrated Treatment is indeed a living art even as healing is a living art. This conscious interaction between two people is an art that arises from the heart and flows through the hands. It should be approached with commitment and concern for positive results.

How incredible it is that we may know where to touch someone's feet and make the person feel better. What a simple healing tool we have available at our fingertips, working in much the same way as radar, scanning the sky for trouble in order to protect.

2

Experience with Pressure-Point Therapy and How It Works

Although it is not necessary, a brief review of the research that has gone into pressure-point therapy and contact healing over the years can be helpful to the reader in understanding how the various schools of application have come into being. It may also give some indication of the direction that healing will take in the future.

To begin with, it is not something new. Pressure-point therapy has been around for a long, long time, and in many different countries of the world. In recent years, however, instruction in the different principles has become available in the United States, making its existence better known. The large amount of publicity that acupuncture, for instance, has had during the past few years has made it more acceptable to the public and more available for research. This same publicity also has had a halo effect over other systems, and we are more aware of the practice of shiatsu, reflexology, and polarity, to name but a few.

When did it all start? And what direction has it taken?

The view of the body as having paths of energy and coordinated reflex points has existed for literally thousands of years. Early Asian civilizations knew about these energy pathways and their correlation with the body functions. Their doctors practiced reflexive treatments for many centuries but more commonly on the smaller areas of the body such as the feet and ears. They recognized at an early date that the body does have pathways of energy and fluids which, when blocked and congested by tension, diet, life style, and environmental insults, lay the body open to disease and unbalanced emotions. It is from this early knowledge that acupuncture, shiatsu, polarity, foot reflexology, and other schools with specialized reflex systems eventually developed. And it is interesting to note that discoveries made in one school were frequently borrowed and incorporated into the study and practice of others.

One of the ancient systems was that of the Japanese *Amma* (*Ampress, Ma-stroke*), the art of rubbing the body and paying particular attention to stiff, tender, and congested areas. No doubt this existed alongside acupuncture for hundreds of years.

Acupuncture was first used in China but was introduced into Japan about 1,300 years ago. This therapy is based on the practice of inserting needles into *tsubos* of the body to relieve pain and suffering in organs that relate to the tsubos. Tsubos, by the way, are nothing more than loci of acu-points located throughout the body. There are 365 major tsubos that run throughout the 14 main meridians, or pathways, of the body. Chi' energy, a life force equal to that which flows through the whole universe, runs along these meridians and can be stimulated and unblocked at these loci points. Different tsubos correspond to different organs. Acupuncture has probably been perfected more in China and Japan than elsewhere. Today it is being practiced more and more in the United States, Russia, and Europe.

Another system closely related to acupuncture is shiatsu. It developed in the eighteenth century in Japan as a combination of Amma massage and acupuncture. It, too, recognizes the 365 tsubos. But instead of using needles, practitioners press the tsubos with their fingers in various ways to achieve a tonifying or stimulating effect on the correlated organs. Another form of shiatsu is called *Azeketsu* therapy. In this system any place where there is pain or tenderness is regarded as a tsubo, and it is stimulated with the thumbs.

The basis of both acupuncture and shiatsu is chi' and the recognition that chi' must be kept free-flowing in its pathways of the body to maintain balance and health.

The recognition of the importance of unobstructed energy flow is also the basis of another system called "zone therapy."

A Connecticut medical doctor, William H. Fitzgerald, was the first to discover zone therapy in the United States, early in the twentieth century. An ear, nose, and throat specialist, he correlated the zones on the body with zones of the feet, the hands, and the face. Then by pressing certain hand and foot reflexes, and using constriction and stimulation with rubber bands and metallic combs, he discovered he was able to produce the effect of anesthesia. This he used on his patients while performing minor surgery.

Another medical doctor, Edwin R. Bowers of New York, studied under Fitzgerald and while writing an article about the therapy gave it its name. Drs. Fitzgerald and Bowers jointly wrote about this new pressure-point system in a book which divided the body into five longitudinal zones on each of the right and the left sides of the body. Thus there were ten zones in this system. By pressing certain points within one zone, one is able to affect other bodily parts and organs lying within that zone. For example, the first zone passes through the thyroid area and the big toe. Fitzgerald found that by pressing the base of the big toe he could affect and stimulate the thyroid and parathyroid.

Another who came to specialize in this area was George Starr White, M.D., of California, who worked with Fitzgerald and Bowers and who added to a revision of their book.

Fitzgerald had been concerned primarily with longitudinal zones. In 1919 a Dr. Joe Shelby Riley published in a book titled *Zone Therapy Simplified* his own discovery of corresponding horizontal zones of the feet while at the same time confirming Fitzgerald's longitudinal lines.

Fitzgerald will be remembered as the one who first described zone therapy as "reflexology," and he and Bowers together were the real pioneers in reflexology in this country. In 1924 Joe Shelby Riley and W. E. Daglesh co-authored a book on zone reflexology, which further developed the reflexive zones.

Still others have contributed to the growth in knowledge and public use of this healing system. Eunice D. Ingham Stopfel and her student Mildred Carter have both written successful, lay-oriented works that have reached and inspired many people.

And not to be forgotten is the Japanese psychologist, Dr. Krura-kichi Hirata, who, even before Fitzgerald, located twelve horizon-tal zones which contained reflex points to the twelve body zones.

By the mid-1900's a new study was well underway—one that was considerably ahead of its time. With great detail and thoroughness Dr. Randolph Stone described patterns of lines of force which operate throughout the body and which he found to be closely related to the patterns of growth of the human fetus in the womb. His intricate and amazing studies developed the notion that the human body may be thought of as having related negative and pos-itive poles. By stimulating reflex points in terms of these poles, negative blockages can be neutralized, thereby establishing balance within the body. Stone developed adjustments and reflex points for the entire body. He recognized the importance of foot work and the powerful correlation of points on the feet with the entire body and psyche of the human being. He also stressed diet, exercise, and spiritual study. His main student, Pierre Pantier, continues to teach workshops over the entire world. This is called "polarity therapy."

One who has studied the relationship of reflexology and acu-puncture in depth is Dr. Ralph Alan Dale, director of the Acu-puncture Education Center in Florida. He compares and correlates the acupuncture meridians with the reflexive points of the feet and postulates that the meridians are fully represented on small areas of the body, such as on the feet. These areas he labels as "micro-acupuncture" systems, and he refers to his own system as "podo-therapy." His paper on this subject given at the Third World Sym-posium on Acupuncture and Chinese Medicine in New York in March 1975 definitely ties acupuncture and reflexology together. We may expect to learn more of his interesting work in forthcom-ing papers.

Acupuncture on the foot has been further researched and devel-oped by a Taiwanese, one Ching-Chang Tung, in a current book.

Another reflex system of the foot has been developed in Japan. Called *sokshindo,* it presents twenty-five specific foot reflex points. This system is best described in a book titled *How to Observe Toes*, written by Shibata Watoku, whose son Shibata Sadao has further developed the system and written books recommending it for family health care. Shibata Sadao currently teaches this system in Tokyo, where it is very popular and highly respected.

Earlier we mentioned shiatsu. Since the 1920's this has become very popular in Japan with many people studying shiatsu in two-year schools which have graduated over 20,000 licensed shiatsu therapists. Most are from the Nippon Shiatzu School, run by Tokujiro Namikoshi. His system specifies forty-four points on the feet alone, not to mention the other tsubos located throughout the body.

A few years ago Watau Ohashi opened his Shiatsu Dojo (institute) in New York, teaching various kinds of pressure-point therapy and reflexology as well as shiatsu. His recent book, *Do-It-Yourself Shiatsu*, teaches the therapist to prevent discomfort, heal, and maintain health by pressing on certain parts of the body including the feet.

In recent years there have been other researchers who have studied and verified the correlation between the feet and the body. One, a Belgian chiropractor, Dr. H. Gillet, has successfully written about such correlations through ten editions of his book, *Belgian Chiropractic Research Notes*. His experiments have proven that the spine and the feet do indeed have direct correlations. The toes correspond to the upper cervical vertebrae, the metatarsals to the other cervical vertebrae, and the tarsal-metatarsal joints to the thoracic vertebrae. This verifies and complies with the zones of many other reflexologists and doctors.

He also revealed that the metatarsal fixations (blockages between joints) correspond to fixations between the ribs themselves, and the spine and the ribs. He proved that by working the feet, by correcting bone articulations (joints), and by limbering stimulation, he had corresponding results with the spine. Instruments proved this reciprocity between the feet and spine, that by working and releasing blocks on one, the same are released on the other.

Dr. Lindberg, an American chiropractor, found a direct relationship between the talus bone of the foot and its joint with adjacent bones, to the fifth lumbar vertebrae of the spine. Thus, when one does a plexus pull and ankle rotation as taught in the basic integrated foot treatment presented in this book, one directly affects and releases the lower back as well as the nerves to the genitals and lower parts of the body.

Recently, with scientific perseverance and technology, many validations of these reflexive systems have been possible. A French medical doctor, Paul Nogier, for instance, has researched the ancient science of diagnosis and treatment of the body by points on the ear (auriculotherapy). His 1975 paper titled "Treatise of Auriculotherapy" presents sound scientific physical evidence.

Dr. Dale too is doing a most exciting and important work based on Motyama's computerized acupuncture instruments to measure and record the main meridians of the human body. This enables him to validate scientifically a direct relationship between the reflex points on the feet with acupuncture points on the body. This gives scientific proof to bolster experimental evidence that foot reflexology works.

Dale's experiments also proved that foot reflex points are useful in both diagnosis and treatment when he concluded that "It is possible to identify meridian and organ pathology with two minutes of foot palpation." This could be done by using fingers, needles, heat, electricity, or any other type of instrument; and it was found to be equally effective when one examines one's own feet.

In Korea, too, the finding of physical proof of acupuncture meridians has been claimed by Professor Kim Bong Han and his staff. They have found a physical system (called *kyungrak*) of integrated ducts, which Dr. Han says are pathways for the meridians. These pathways are filled with a fluid he calls *sanal*. Sanal contains DNA, RNA, and protein and is somehow involved with cell formation. While his duct theory also substantiates the meridian theory, it further reveals how treatment through pressure or needles directly affects the healing of the patient.

The Soviet Union has completely accepted Han's work. In fact Russian scientists have continually researched, respected, and used alternative healing methods since first beginning their studies early this century. Russia is the only country having free, government-sponsored fasting centers that maintain detailed records of the results. In Russia today, acupuncture is completely validated, approved, and accepted; it is used daily in coordination with Western medical methods. Since 1968, respected Soviet scientists have pub-

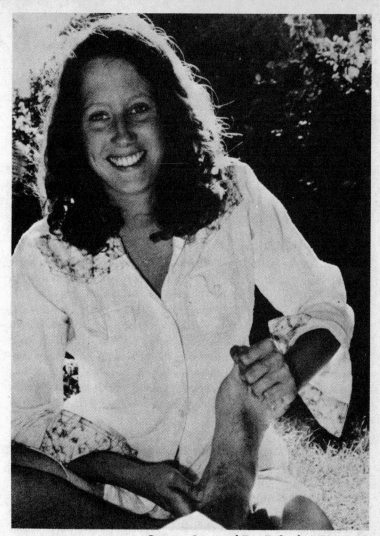

Giving an Integrated Foot Reflexology Treatment.

licly stated that all living things have a physical body and a counter-
part energy body, and that physical healing can take place by
dealing with this energy body.

And finally, in China today acupuncture courses are mandatory
in medical schools.

What all this says is that these methods have been proved to
work through experience and are now being proved to work scientifically. While more research is obviously needed to understand

them completely, their efficacy, which has been known through practice for centuries, cannot be denied.

While we know that pressure on a specific point will obtain a positive reaction in another part of the body related to the specific point, we still have trouble answering the question, "How does it happen; what are the precise mechanisms?"

At this moment in history, no one can answer this question with complete satisfaction. But perhaps because of the research presently going on, we may one day find the answer coming from one or more of the following major theories:

- Professor Han's *kyungrak* theory of the existence of sanal ducts, which are the paths of meridians. He postulates that stimulating acupressure tsubos is a direct way to stimulate sanal, which, in turn, affects our bodies on the cellular and germinal levels.
- C. C. Gunn, F. G. Ditchburn, M. H. Hing, and G. J. Renwick, all medical doctors, published a neurological explanation of acupuncture in a 1976 *American Journal of Chinese Medicine*. Testing acupoints with a neurometer, they found that all tsbuos contain a rich supply of superficial nerves. They believe that orthodox medicine will accept the validity of this type of therapy if the acupuncture points are renamed and studied as points of direct nerve stimulation.
- Dr. Cesar Mishann Pinto, M.D., Professor of Surgery and Chairman of the General Hospital of Guatemala, postulates that stimulation of the acupressure tsubos directly affects the lymphatics and by this affects specific organs and the entire body.
- The School of Applied Kinesiology (Dr. Goodheart, D.C. and Dr. Walther, D.C.) regard foot reflexes as proprioceptive nerve receptors, receptors which send impulses to all parts of the body, as to Golgi tendon and muscle spindle cells.
- There are many theories based on the assumption that the body is a network of energy pathways and that stimulation of the tsubos will release energy blockages and restore balances. As of now these theories do not satisfy the Western mind as to the step-by-step procedure by which rebalancing occurs.
- Another theory is concerned with lactic acid. It is said that reflex treatments can release up to 80 per cent of the lactic acid resi-

dues in the body, allowing it to flow back to the liver to be recycled as glycogen, or energy.

- There are those who believe that the muscles store repressed psychological inhibitions and tensions, which, when pressure points are stimulated, mechanically release the psychological stress that prevents both bodily and emotional balance.

Whatever the outcome of future research, it is obvious that re-flexology does work and is a tool that should be known to everyone. Although we cannot pinpoint the mechanisms, we can reap the results. Why shouldn't we touch someone and rid him or her of a headache, a stiff neck, or a depression even though we cannot explain the therapy mechanism? Why need we look only to lifeless pills or uncompassionate syrups and potions when we can reach out through our concern and touch to restore peace and balance?

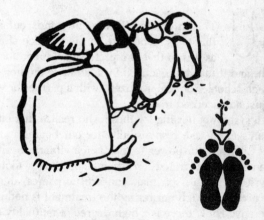

3

The Integrated Treatment: Preparation and Exploration

The Integrated Treatment stands out as a system that is as responsive to the practice of a lay person as it is to that of a professional practitioner. It is not difficult, and it may be practiced by a father or mother, husband or wife, high schooler or senior citizen, with a partner or without one, or by just a concerned friend.

It is a system of healing for those who realize that our wise Creator wants us to take responsibility for our bodies and minds and has put it within our power to maintain a vibrant, healthy body.

Because the Integrated Treatment approaches foot reflexology on physical, mental, spiritual, and artistic planes, the satisfaction one receives while administering the treatment is nothing less than self-therapy. Thus, there is a high degree of mutuality on the parts of both practitioner and patient.

So, the system is for those who want to heal and achieve the optimum balance for themselves as well as for others.

How, then, does one learn this treatment and use this book? It is best if we think in terms of preparation and exploration before we get into basic strokes and techniques.

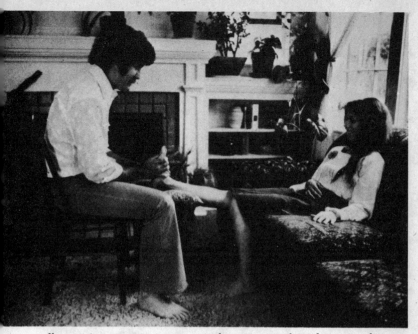

You can give a treatment to someone who is sitting up, lying down, or reclining, as long as you both are comfortable.

Preparation

POSITIONS

The patient may lie down, sit in a chair, or even prop himself partly up. The important thing is that you must be able to work on the feet with freedom of movement.

Make sure you are both relaxed. Tension in your body can transfer to your patient.

Your body and the patient's should be comfortable, the hands and legs of your partner not crossed, for that blocks the free flow of energy currents. (In fact, if you are ever in a threatening situation and wish to remove yourself from its energies but cannot leave the room, cross your legs at the knees and fold your arms in front of you. This maintains an energy separation between you and another person. But in treatment, avoid separation as much as possible.)

Advise the patient to let go completely when you touch or move him. He must not help you; he must be encouraged to relax and enjoy the treatment. With shoes and socks removed, the feet may rest on a clean towel.

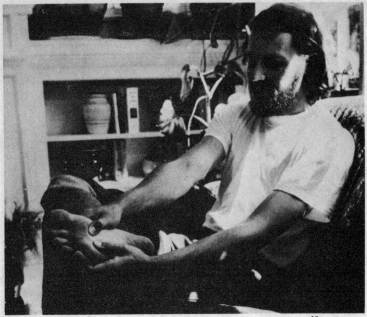
Giving a self-treatment.

SELF-POSITION

When performing a treatment on yourself, you have several positions to choose. You may sit in a chair or on the floor with one foot high on the opposite thigh. You may also find it very satisfying to sit on the edge of a bathtub, soaking one foot in the water or under running water while working on the other foot, which rests on your other thigh. Running water is high in energy and stimulates the body's circulation, the nervous system, and body vibrations.

SETTING THE SCENE

Health is a state of ease, and the more relaxed a person is, the more healing can take place. If there is time, try to arrange a scene that promotes peace. Even when alone, it is good to surround yourself in a relaxing atmosphere. Soft lights or candles create a helpful mood. So do soft words, meditation, and breathing exercises. So does washing your patient's feet. (For footbaths, see Appendix of Oils, Creams, Packs, and Footbaths.)

If cramped for time, a treatment can be given anywhere; but unless the treatment is given just for purposes of relaxation, it is best to have no music (which can distract you). Incessant chatter is bad. Beware of interruptions. Disconnect the phone before you begin.

As for yourself, don't let your hands leave the feet or break contact once you have begun the treatment. You should have no long nails that can stick and hurt the skin.

Finally, since blood is drawn away from the extremities to go to the digestive organs after eating, delay any treatment until at least two hours after the patient has eaten. Otherwise both digestion and treatment will become diluted and impaired.

WHAT TO TELL THE PATIENT

Instill confidence in him by explaining what you are doing.

Encourage questions anytime. And encourage the patient to tell you how he feels.

Explain that the treatment is a process of cleansing the body. It releases blocked energy. It releases toxins and accumulated wastes, which are absorbed back into the bloodstream to be later eliminated by the kidneys and liver. Before such elimination, however, the patient may temporarily experience headaches, nausea, diarrhea, or a cold. This is part of the cleansing process on the road to better health. Assure the patient that each person may react to treatment in different ways, some with immediate feelings of renewed health, and some with little or delayed reactions.

Encourage your patient to tell you which strokes feel especially good, and which ones hurt; for you do not wish to hurt. (Eventually you will become adept at detecting pain via your fingertips.)

CONTACT

Your hands should be relaxed and warm. A few simple exercises for this are shaking them hard and then stretching them out as far as possible; folding the hands together and squeezing them hard; stretching each finger by pulling with the opposite hand and hold-

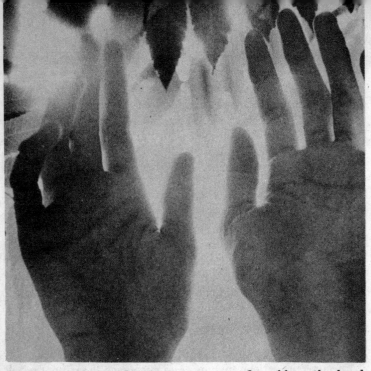

ing the stretch for fifteen or twenty seconds; rubbing the hands with the knuckles of the opposite hand; and squeezing tennis balls or paper balls.

But if they are still cold, hold them under warm running water. This will stimulate the flow of energy currents and renew the energy field around the body. Hands should always be washed before and after treatments.

Before touching the patient, rub your hands together until you feel heat; then gently lower them to the patient's feet, being aware of passing them through the energy zone which surrounds his body. Notice how it feels to penetrate this zone.

Now touch the feet slowly. *The first contact is often the most important contact, for it influences the whole treatment.* Hold the feet a few minutes while you orient yourself and allow the patient to become used to your close contact. Then work right on the skin without oil, which gets in the way and blocks energy transfer.

Exploration

Once the feet are in your hands, begin to explore. This is not a part of the Integrated Treatment, but a time for you, when first learning massage, to develop a comfortable and sensitive touch. While you do this, keep this book by your side. Switch off between periods of exploring to check the charts at the front and rear of the book to identify what you see and feel. And explore, too, with closed eyes to get a "feel" for the sensitivity of your touch and the quality of life beneath your fingers. Guidelines for exploration are:

- Take time to become acquainted with the feet.
- Experience how bone feels under skin.
- Experience how muscles feel.
- Feel the difference in tone between muscles and tendons.
- Feel the difference in temperature on the different areas of the feet (good health should reveal even temperatures).
- Feel the difference in texture on the different areas of the skin.
- Feel the feet with different parts of your hand: the palm, top of hand, nails, individual fingers.
- Learn the differences in the sensitivities of your ten fingers.

Close your eyes and explore.

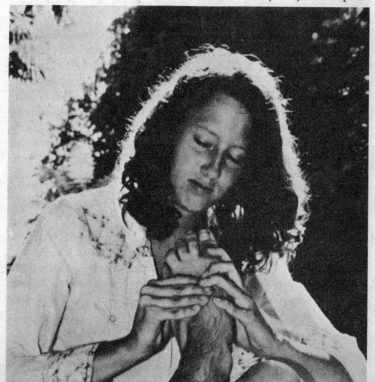

- Be aware of soft areas and hard areas. Press the feet lightly, then hard. Use this time to become comfortable with skin, muscles, bone, tendons, and ligaments.
- With pressure from your thumbs, focus on feeling:
  - A healthy resiliency. This means everything is fine.
  - A hard resistance. This means there is tension, deposits, or degeneration (unless you are feeling a normal ligament, tendon, or bone; check the charts).
  - A hollow or recessed area without resiliency. This means lack of nutrition and energy blockages.
  Note: The latter two areas need pressure therapy stimulation.

There are certain exercises that develop the sensitivity of fingers. Close your eyes and try to feel a thread that has been placed under the page of a book. Try it again under two pages. Keep putting the thread under yet another page until you no longer feel it. Do this daily, trying each time to feel the thread through more and more paper. Try it also with dental floss, different widths of rubber bands, and with seeds of different sizes. Try outlining leaves and flowers under paper with your fingers, searching for all details. Then draw what you were able to feel and compare the drawing with the actual object.

Developing sensitive fingers is a must for the practitioner. The artful healer, which is the goal of the Integrated Treatment system, uses his or her hands as though creating a living sculpture. Through practice you can become sensitive to the incredible radarlike potential of your fingertips. All living cells have a cellular intelligence of their own. Your hands are intelligent and can feel and receive much more than you would ever guess.

Practice conveying with your hands confidence, comfort, and constancy (a flowing rhythm). Take your time and pay attention to details because the patient is rediscovering his or her body, too, through your fingertips.

Caution: Do not give a treatment if you feel ill or in low energy. At such times it is impossible to channel energy to another person; and you can actually drain energy from another by trying to give a treatment under such circumstances. Under normal conditions, however, there is a long-lasting exchange of energy; so let's hope you may give many treatments to those people whose vibrations you would like to carry around.

4

The Integrated Treatment: Basic Strokes

In this chapter we shall be concerned with the strokes a practitioner uses to manipulate, or work, the foot. All strokes stimulate blood flow and nerve nourishment. However, different strokes have specialized effects. We shall describe these strokes and their specific purposes.

BASIC SWEDISH MASSAGE MOVEMENTS

Effleurage. This is a firm pressure to assist venous and lymphatic drainage toward the heart.

Petrissage. A stimulating, kneading movement in several forms, much like kneading bread or stretching in circular movements. It stimulates muscular and nervous structures. By stretching adipose (fatty) tissue, it releases toxins stored there. And many toxins, pesticides, and additives have an amazing affinity for fat cells.

Friction. Larger petrissage movements, to stimulate broader muscle structure of the body.

Tapotement. Use of the fists, or cupped palms, or the loose flinging of the hands to percuss a body area. Best done parallel to the muscle fibers to prevent trauma and spasm.

BASIC POLARITY MOVEMENTS

Stimulation. Placing a finger or hand on one contact and holding it there, yet moving it back and forth gently. Not a rubbing movement. This speeds up the flow of energy current to the related organ and system.

Massage. Placing the finger or hand on a point and rubbing over a larger area of the skin, thus contacting a number of points. Massage may be done in vertical, horizontal, or circular movements.

SHIATSU MOVEMENTS

Acupressure. Therapeutic pressure with the fingers, especially the thumbs, on specific meridian points. This pressure corrects irregularities in the flow of chi' energy, releases excess lactic acid in the fibers (commonly known as "stiffness"), and improves the general tone, resistance, and repair of the body.

Pressure Specific. Using a ball-point pen, the point hidden inside the pen, to apply very specific pressure to a tiny area, such as the corner near a toe nail.

INTEGRATED REFLEXOLOGY STROKES

Reflex point. Very similar to acupressure loci except that the reflex point is based both on points on reflex zones and points on meridian pathways. Pressing of the reflex point may be done in these three ways:

1. By massaging, or rubbing the general area of the reflex point, searching for the tenderest spot, deposits, resistance, or "dull hollows." When you find such points, *apply constant, firm pressure on them with the ball or tip of your thumb.* Release pressure after five to fifteen seconds, or when the tenderness leaves, or when you feel an increase in energy flow, experienced like a pulse beat starting up. This pulsation signifies a release of the blocked energy. It is important to become sensitive to the lack and presence of this pulsation at reflex points.

2. By *inching*, or moving the thumb, bit by bit, along a specific area. This is a combination of applying pressure each time the ball and then the tip of the thumb contacts the skin. It is similar to a caterpillar's inching its way along, and presses numerous points in a short time.

3. By finding the contact, pressing with the ball of your thumb and stimulating the contact. This means *keeping the thumb on the one contact but rubbing back and forth gently.* Find the reflex point by working the areas labeled on Charts I and II. Since reflex areas vary from person to person, it is best to work the general area and search for the most tender or granular spot. That becomes the reflex point most important to stimulate.

Breath stroke. The breath itself is used as a stroke. You can actually direct your breath to an area to help heal it. The ancients recognized this and emphasized breathing techniques for relaxation and healing. So do we. Science, too, has proven that breathing has great control over our bodies and our minds. The mind tends to follow the breath; so by slowing down the breath we can slow down and control our minds. Through repeated practice and visualization, you can learn to direct your breath to any part of the body—yours or your patient's—to heighten the effect of stimulating a reflex. Your psyche follows your mind, which follows your breath, so directed breath focuses the potential healing energy of the psyche to the reflex, too.

When you take a breath, make sure it is deep: fill up the lower rib cage, then chest, and then upper chest. This is referred to as three-part deep breathing. When you exhale, exhale deeply in the reverse order. Guide your patient if he or she needs help.

The breath stroke is done in three steps:

1. Guide your patient to "Inhale." Both of you take a deep breath and direct it to the organ that corresponds to the reflex under your finger. When inhaling, both practitioner and patient should feel that oxygen, vitality, life and health are being drawn to the area.

2. Guide your patient to "Exchange." Explain that you both now concentrate on the good elements in the breath replacing the bad, degenerating cells in the organ, making an exchange of health for disease.

3. Guide your patient to "Exhale" and both of you mentally command the organ to "Release and Relax!" For example, "Stomach, Release and Relax!" or "Heal and Relax!"

In short then:

Inhale—controlling breath to a specific spot.
Exchange—concentrating on positive replacing negative.
Exhale—releasing of negativity from body and giving a mental command.

The patient should be encouraged to continue this on his own at home, with problem organs.

You can press reflex points
in the following manners:

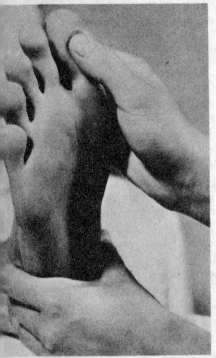

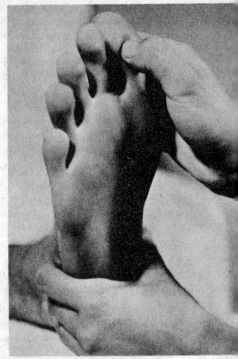

Pressing with the flat ball of the thumb.

Pressing with the tip of the thumb.

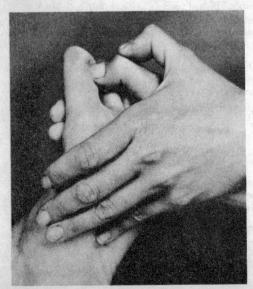

One thumb supporting the other.

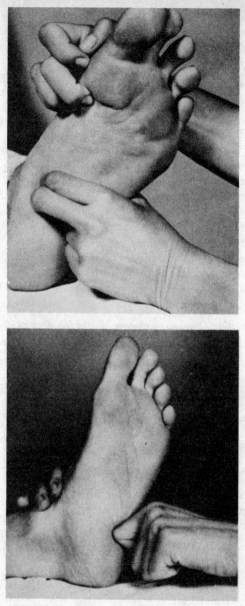

Pressing with other convenient fingers.

Pressing with the knuckle.

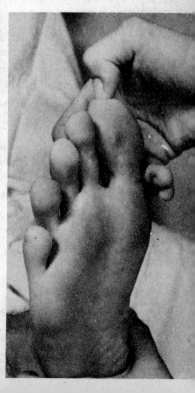

Inching with the nail.

Visualization stroke. This is one of the most important strokes to understand and practice, because it is so powerful. It is a stroke in which you visualize energy pouring in and through you, out of your hands and into your patient.

Visualize a flow of liquid sunlight, if you will, being poured into the top of your head. Not easy? No, but a little practice will help you visualize whatever you wish. Visualizing what you wish to have happen is such a successful tool that it is used by literally thousands of salesmen to increase their orders, by people who are trying to break old habits and build new ones, by ministers, doctors, and just about everyone imaginable because it is so powerful in obtaining the results one wants.

So with the Integrated Treatment, we use a visualization of energy pouring through our body and into the patient, with the knowledge that this really draws healing energy into their bodies. This stroke may be outlined as follows:

- "See" and feel the warm, liquid flow of energy pour into the top of your head, down your neck, through your arms.
- "See" and feel the flow pour from your hands into the foot reflex.
- "See" and feel the flow pour deeper into the patient's body, directed to the specific organ you are stimulating.

Once adept at visualization, you can experience a tingling, warm feeling, often accompanied by a humming sound, and a strong sense of channeling energy. Keep the visualization centered throughout the massage for the psychic background it produces. Use it whenever you find a trouble spot.

Do encourage the patient to visualize with you. This is most important, for sharing is always more powerful when energies are combined than when working alone.

Do you believe and want to be healed? So be it. You are healed.

Do you believe you can be a channel for healing? So be it. You are a healer.

Affirmation stroke. This bears a relationship to the visualization stroke. It plants a positive projection of your mind and inner energy in the patient. As you press the reflex point, say to yourself mentally, "This organ (which I am pressing) is being healed."

Nerve stroke. This is one of the final strokes, a very subtle stroke working on subtle levels. It cools the body, gently stimulating the nerve fiber endings and ends of meridian pathways and clearing negative energy clinging about the body. It is done rapidly and gently by moving the hands along the body in a sweeping manner, the hands just touching the small hairs and not the skin. If well done, it often causes slight goose bumps, and is very refreshing.

Final cleansing stroke. This is the same as the nerve stroke but done two to three inches away from the body. It cleans the electrical corona around the body of residual tension and negativity.

Release movements. This refers to any stretch of the tendons and joints, done in this manner:

- Stretch the area to its *fullest "edge"* so to speak.
- Maintain the stretch for a prolonged period of time (usually fifteen to thirty seconds).
- Then stretch *a little beyond* the "edge."
- Then release.

Tendons are pathways for electromagnetic current. Any good stretch of the tendons releases energy and clears the pathways.

By maintaining the stretch and tension of the muscle, nutrition and oxygen gush in. Fibers are limbered. The stretch also pulls embedded toxins out of adipose tissue. Shallow, bouncy stretches back and forth do little good; they should be progressive and prolonged.

As you do all the strokes, you are always on the lookout for: areas of resistance, pain, unhealthy hollows, and hardened, granular deposits. All these areas require special attention. What you feel as granular deposits may be:

- Undissolved acids, such as lactic or uric, due to trauma, overuse, lack of nutrition or oxygen, and poor circulation.
- Injured, hardened, or inflamed nerve fiber endings.
- Tension or energy blocks.

- Tissue degeneration and hardening from lack of nutrition in the area, due to poor circulation, to trauma, etc. This results in constant contraction, which results in hardening and even possible death at the cellular level. This condition may be likened to mini-adhesions or tiny scabs inside the foot.
- Pollutants, foreign particles, metallic build-up, toxins directed to the feet by gravity, and/or fatty accumulations such as cholesterol.
- Fatty deposits that have solidified or become fibrous. I have seen for myself, in dissection of human cadavers, arteries with cholesterol and fatty deposits that have become so hardened they will actually produce a *cling* sound when tapped with a scalpel. Diet, exercise, and treatments could have eliminated these.
- Calcifications and spurs in abnormal areas such as muscle.
- Manifestation of an aberrant proprioceptive nerve receptor arc.

Foot treatments can dissolve and release these problems. Work each reflex for each corresponding organ as shown on Charts I, II, and III. Individuals vary in the placement of each reflex to slight degrees, so be flexible and search and stimulate.

Frequently you will find very tender spots. Apply pressure with your thumb until the patient experiences a "good hurt," which is pressure that may be comfortably tolerated. Most people can tolerate twenty to twenty-five pounds of pressure. (Practicing by pressing the bathroom scale will give you help in estimating pressure.) Some people can tolerate a lot, others little—tune in to each individual. Hold this pressure until you feel a healthy, rhythmic pulsation, or until the patient feels a release. This means that the pain is gone although the pressure is still felt. You may now release the reflex, stimulate the spot a few times. Always repeat this two more times before going on to the next point.

When reflex points are especially painful, return to them frequently during the treatment rather than staying with them too long at one time. This way you will not bruise the area and break tiny capillaries and the patient will not become tense (the face will indicate that).

Why are reflex points tender? They are always more tender than the organs themselves; being on currents that flow through the body, they are affected by energy blockages to all organs on that current. Often they are five to twenty times more sensitive than the organ itself.

Throughout treatments, make good use of your thumbs, for they are more sensitive than other fingers. Or, if your thumbs get tired, first locate the tender spots with the thumb; then continue working with other fingers or with knuckles. Continued use will strengthen the thumb; until then you may wish to use a thumb-on-thumb technique for additional pressure. Like a runner, thumbs and fingers have a "second wind," so stick with it during any low ebbs, and any tiredness will disappear.

SUMMARY

Pressing the pressure points on the patient also affects you. Your fingertips are connected to the brain. Using your hands and pressing your fingers promotes your own physiological stability and health. That portion of your brain going to your hands is larger than any other specific portion of the brain. You also have numerous spinal nerves feeding your hands—more to your hands than to any other part of your body. Every time you press, you activate all that spinal energy. As you touch, you, too, are being touched.

5

The Integrated Treatment: Basic Techniques and Procedures

First we suggest an outline of steps to follow. You may omit, add, or you may change the order. You are encouraged to learn these steps thoroughly so you will have a good foundation for your own style.

These steps are built upon the basic strokes of Chapter 4 with certain variations.

The basic treatment should take about a half hour to forty-five minutes once you become comfortable and agile with the strokes.

Remember always to use breath and visualization strokes whenever you find particularly deep tension, pain, or other trouble.

You are urged to make frequent use of the foot charts that appear on the endpapers of this book. Study these charts carefully before giving any treatment and first practice locating the specific areas on your own feet. More detailed illustrations will accompany much of the explanatory text.

Always begin with the right foot.

The Basic Treatment

STEP 1: OPENING

1. Rub hands briskly till warm and slowly lower them onto the feet.
2. The patient takes five deep breaths.
3. As he or she exhales, instruct them to make a mental command to "Relax!"
4. While he does this, hold both solar plexus reflexes (located just below the lung area in Chart I) with each thumb. The rest of your fingers rest on the tops of the feet. Either do a breathing stroke on him or use this time to do your affirmations and visualizations.

Pressing both solar plexus reflexes while the patient takes five deep breaths.

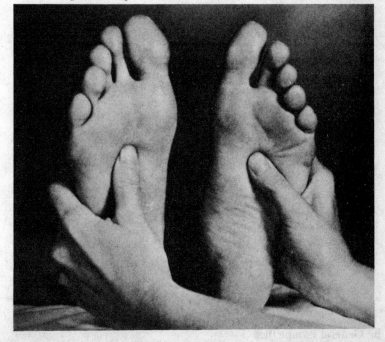

STEP 2: GENERAL MOVEMENTS

1. Beginning effleurage
2. Wringing stroke
3. Lymphatic effleurage
4. Top of foot stimulation
5. Bottom of foot stimulation
6. Tendon stretch

STEP 3: ANKLE MOVEMENTS

1. Flexion and extension releases, lateral and medial stretch, rotation
2. Plexus pull
3. Flexion and extension against resistance
4. Tendon-notch stimulation
5. Ankle points
6. Effleurage of ankle

STEP 4: TOE STROKES

1. Circular petrissage, lateral petrissage
2. Toe release, toe pull with tendon stimulation
3. Rotation
4. Flexion and extension release
5. Big toe adjustment
6. Reflex points
7. Nail-inching
8. Base stretch
9. Toe effleurage

STEP 5: SPECIFICS

1. Points on the sole of the foot
2. Points for the lateral (outside) foot
3. Points for the medial (inside) foot
4. Points on the top of the foot
5. Points on the leg:
   a. Friction
   b. Inside shin points
   c. Stomach 36 and lateral calf points
   d. Center calf points
6. General Lymphatics

STEP 6: CLOSING

1. Tapotement
2. Venous pump
3. Final effleurage
4. Nerve stroke
5. Final cleansing

STEP 7: REPEAT THE ABOVE SIX STEPS ON THE LEFT FOOT.

STEP 8: HEALING AFFIRMATION

With this outline in mind, we shall now perform this basic treatment. You are reminded that all effleurage and rotation strokes should be done at least three times. We shall start with Step 2 since Step 1 has already been explained.

STEP 2: GENERAL MOVEMENTS

1. *Beginning effleurage.* Step 1: Mold your hands to the contour of the top of the foot. With firm pressure (about twenty-five pounds), make an upward stretching stroke to the knee. If the leg has a lot of hair, press up the leg every few inches in a pumping rather than stretching manner. This is more desirable than getting your fingers slippery. Step 2: Mold hand to back of calf and lightly (five pounds pressure) come down to Achilles tendon. Pull it firmly downward (twenty pounds pressure) stretching the heel out well. Step 3: Place your thumbs on the sole of the foot and your fingers on the top; stretch the sole from the heel upward to the toes. This entire movement should be done in one flowing stroke, up the front of the leg, down the back including the Achilles heel, and up the foot.

   Throughout the treatment, effleurage should follow every variation of petrissage. Petrissage releases toxins, and effleurage encourages the bloodstream to hurry them off to the sewage plant of the liver and kidneys. Effleurage in small areas is just a firm rubbing of that spot toward the heart.

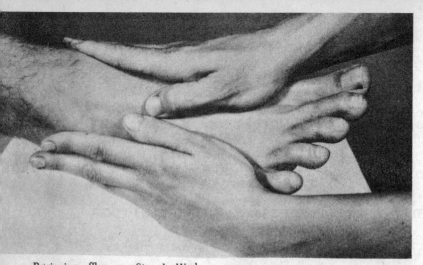

Beginning effleurage, Step 1. Work
up to the knee.

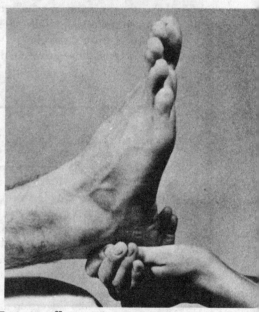

Beginning effleurage, Step 2. Down
the calf, and stretch heel.

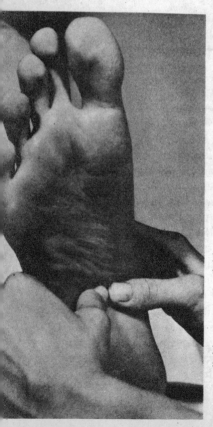

Beginning effleurage, Step 3. Stretch
sole up to toes.

2. **Wringing stroke.** Basically a friction movement. Grab hold of the foot just as you would a sponge you wish to wring dry, one hand above the other. Wring and twist your hands in opposite directions, firmly and slowly. Do this up and down the foot from ankle to toes. Use as much steady pressure as the patient can handle.

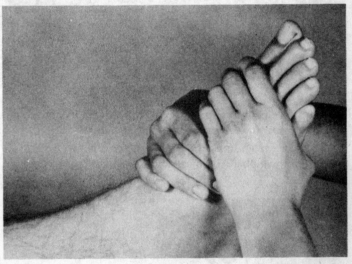

Wringing stroke.

This is one of the most delightful strokes. When done properly, patients often request that it be repeated.

3. **Lymphatic effleurage.** There are a number of lymphatic reflex points and movements. Any of them can be used, or in conditions of infection, swelling and congestion, all of them can be successfully used in the following convenient outline: 1. Stimulate the lymphatic drainage reflex points all along the left ankle junction, shown on Chart II. Press your fingers into the reflexes, while pressing the foot perpendicular to the leg, with your thumbs. 2. Press and stimulate lymphatic point between big and second toe, as shown on Chart II. 3. Using your thumb, stretch the skin from the heel along the outside of the foot (the lymphatic reflex region) upward toward the toes. When you reach beneath the little toe, continue the stretch toward the big toe, at the base of all the toes, including the big toe. Use twenty

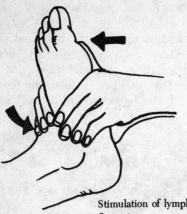

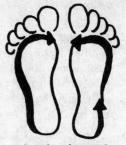

Stretching lymphatic reflexes.

Stimulation of lymphatic drainage reflex points.

to twenty-five pounds of pressure. 4. Finish with General Lymphatics movement (see under Step 5: Specifics).

This stroke may be used after any other effleurage stroke to increase the lymphatic drainage and detoxification process.

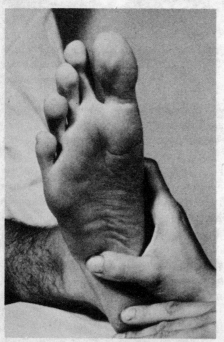

Lymphatic effleurage.

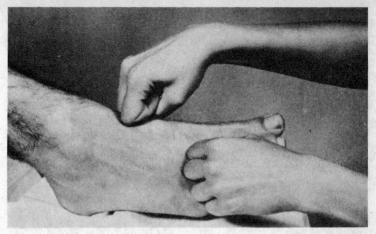

Top of foot stimulation.

4. **Top of foot stimulation.** With your knuckles rapidly rub the top of the foot including the sides, ankles, and toes. When properly done, the patient will feel tingling throughout the entire foot.
5. **Bottom of foot stimulation.** With knuckles, rapidly rub the sole of the foot to stimulate all the points, the nerve and meridian endings and to activate the muscle fibers.

   Top and bottom of foot stimulation may be done simultaneously using one hand on top and the other on the bottom, sandwiching the foot in between.
6. **Tendon stretch.** Each toe has a tendon. Starting at the head end of the foot (the toe end), and beginning with the big toe tendon, use your thumb to stretch the tendon in the direction of the ankle, up into the lymphatic area. One by one, do the other toes; then the spaces in between. Next inch the thumb between the tendons.

Stretching up between the tendons, after stretching the tendons themselves.

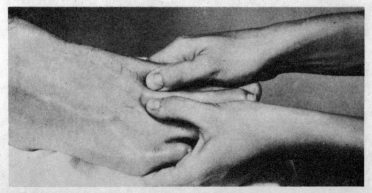

STEP 3: ANKLE MOVEMENTS

1. *Flexion release.* With one hand anchoring the heel and with the palm of the other hand against the sole of the foot, firmly and gently push the foot all the way back (toes and foot toward body) to the edge of the patient's limit. Hold this for fifteen to thirty seconds; then make a good release by pushing a bit further before letting go.

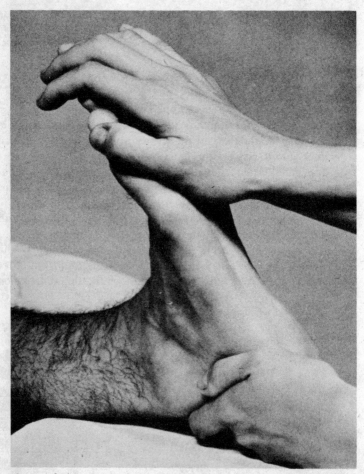

Flexion release.

Extension release. With one hand anchoring the heel and the other on top of the foot, press foot downward as far as it will go (toes and foot toward floor). Hold for fifteen to thirty seconds and release.

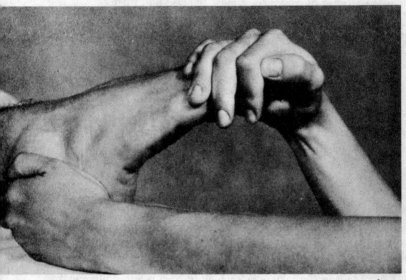

Extension release.

Lateral and medial stretch. Holding the heel with one hand, stretch the foot all the way to the inside (medial). Hold for five to ten seconds and release. Now stretch all the way to the outside (lateral) and hold for five to ten seconds before releasing.

Rotation. With heel well stabilized in one hand, slowly and firmly rotate the foot clockwise with the other. Repeat in a counterclockwise direction.

2. *Plexus pull.* Clasp the fingers of both hands around the top of the foot. The baby fingers should reach the leg at the ankle joint, and thumbs should meet, forming a "V" on the sole of the foot in the plexus region. With a firm clasp, flex the foot up past a right angle with the leg as far as possible, at the same time gently pulling the foot toward you. During this firm flex, the patient should breathe deeply three times. On his last exhalation while you maintain the strong flex, firmly and steadily pull and

jerk the foot straight back toward yourself. This is an adjustment movement which sometimes releases a jammed talus joint. After the jerk, maintain the flex and have the patient take a slow deep breath. Have him hold the breath, then push the solar plexus reflex deeply three times. Release on exhale.

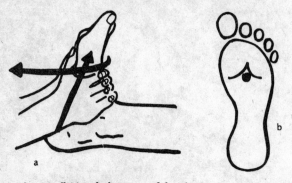

Plexus pull (a) and placement of thumbs (b).

Warn people before you use this stroke that you are going to pull their foot firmly. You may omit it on very sensitive people. This stroke releases tension in the ankle joint and femur and blockages in the talus joints which in turn releases blockages in the fifth lumbar vertebra of the lower back. The stimulation of the solar plexus alerts the subconscious to problems and hidden tensions in the body; thus while you work on reflex points, the subconscious is working, too.

3. *Flexion and extension against resistance.* With the heel in one hand, flex the foot as far as possible with the other. Hold this flexion while patient pushes his foot up and down, slowly, against this resistance. Next extend the foot as far as possible while patient does likewise. This strengthens the lateral or peroneus muscles of the leg, and is an adjustive type movement.

4. *Tendon-notch stimulation.* Place the thumb of one hand into the notch at the top of the foot, at the leg-ankle junction. With the other hand, move the foot, backward into full flexion. This deepens your thumb contact into the notch. Then extend the foot downward while the thumb merely holds the contact, applying no pressure. Continue this, pumping the foot back and forth, pressing and releasing, at least five times.

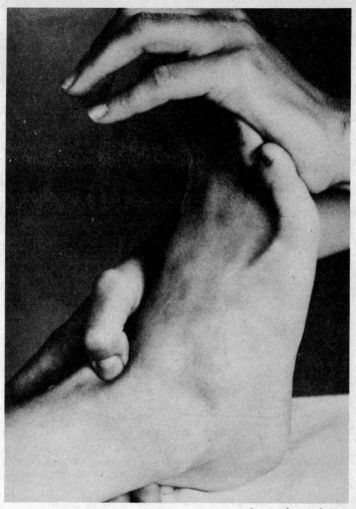

Tendon-notch stimulation.

The tendon notch is a reflex point for the diaphragm and encourages easier breathing. It also stimulates lymphatic flow in the lower extremities and in the upper thorax region.

5. *Ankle points.* Stabilize heel in left hand and press your thumb into reflex points around the ankle. Right hand pumps foot back and forth in flexion and extension. The left thumb deeply presses ankle reflexes on extension only, and lightly holds reflexes in flexion. Repeat this on inside and outside ankle points. Pressure is held three to five seconds, and longer for tender spots.

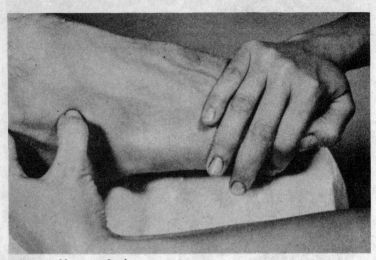

Pressing ankle points firmly on extension.

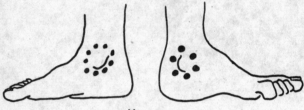

Ankle points.

6. *Effleurage of ankle.* Rub ankle with an upward movement.

STEP 4: TOE STROKES

Each movement may be done on each toe before going on to the next movement, or all may be done on one toe before proceeding to the next. As you work on the toes, firmly stabilize the foot with your free hand.

1. *Circular petrissage.* Starting at the base of the big toe with the thumb on top and the forefinger on the back, make circular stretching movements from the base to the top of the toe while you support the foot with the other hand. Repeat on each toe.

   Lateral petrissage. Starting at the base of the big toe with the thumb on one side and the forefinger on the other, make circu-

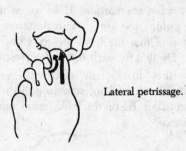

Lateral petrissage.

lar stretching movements from the base to the tip of the toe. Repeat on each toe.

2. *Toe release.* Starting with the big toe, hold the toe close to its base where it comes in contact with the foot, thumb on top where it contacts with the foot, and forefinger on the underside right beneath the joint connecting toe to foot. Support the foot well with the other hand. Pull the toe straight out, not bending the toe downward or upward. Maintain the stretch to the toe's maximum edge for ten seconds followed by a firm jerk straight back to see if you can "crack" the toe. Do not force this. If it does not "crack," forget it and try again later when the foot is more relaxed. Repeat on all toes.

This stimulates all the tendons, releases energy, and clears head and neck congestion. All meridians and nerve endings for the brain and neck regions are stimulated.

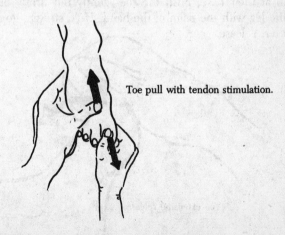

Toe pull with tendon stimulation.

Toe pull with tendon stimulation. Hold toe as described in toe release. While pulling toe firmly, with thumb of the other hand press the tendon of that toe from the toe's base up to the leg-ankle junction. Do this for each toe and corresponding tendon.

3. *Rotation.* Do this firmly, in clockwise and then counterclockwise directions, making sure to pull the toe to the fullest circle it can make. Be on the lookout for sounds, gritty crystals, and resistance.

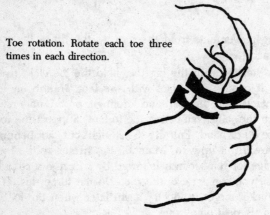

Toe rotation. Rotate each toe three times in each direction.

Rotating the big toe very thoroughly releases neck and shoulder tensions.

4. *Extension release.* With the fingers on top of the toes, pressing in at their base, push the toes gently but firmly back toward the leg with the palm of the hand. Hold stretch, go a little further, release.

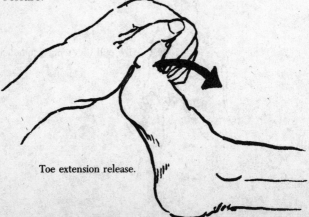

Toe extension release.

Flexion release. Firmly grip the hand over the toes with the thumb resting on top of toes and the fingers underneath in the lung area. Make a quick motion of the entire hand, bending the toes downward and pushing the arch up from underneath by the fingers at the lung reflex.

This movement releases tension in the upper parts of the body, especially the shoulder girdle.

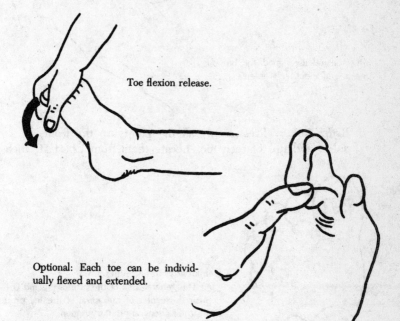

Toe flexion release.

Optional: Each toe can be individually flexed and extended.

5. *Big toe adjustment.* Hold the big toe with one hand and firmly pull it away from the other toes in the direction of the other foot. While holding the big toe, smack the side of the upper thoracic reflex (where the bone sticks out under the toe.) Smack with the fleshy pad of the side of your hand, under the thumb.

This is excellent for bunion problems and should be done five times daily in coordination with a good diet, to help correct this problem. It also helps tight shoulder blades, and clearing the head in the neck, throat, eye, and ear areas.

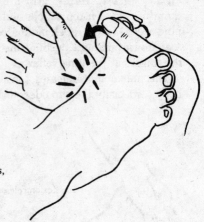

Big toe release, good for bunions, neck, and shoulder problems.

6. **Reflex points.** Press firmly all the points on the front, back, sides, and tips of each toe. Locate them from Chart II. Inch

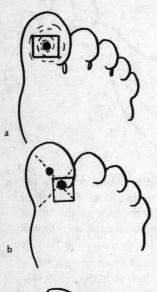

Helpful ways to find reflexes:

(a) The general area of the pituitary gland is in or near the center of the spiral of the toe print. Box signifies general pituitary region.

(b) The pineal gland is about a 45-degree angle downward toward the outer side of the base of the big toe. Divide this line in half, and this is the specific point. Box signifies general pineal region. Thus, look in this area for most tender point.

(c) Gently pull and hold the toes back, enabling fingers to come straight down onto the eye and ear points at the base of the toes, and the thyroid and parathyroid at the base of the big toe.

your thumb down all five zones of the big toe from the tip to its base, one zone at a time. These five zones correspond to all five zones of the head. Stimulate the web of each toe with your thumb and forefinger, front and back. Move the forefinger in and out between the toes, rotating your finger at the same time. As you do this, stabilize and support the toes with your opposite hand.

This is very effective for the eyes, ears, and sinuses. It also feels great, but be a bit more gentle between the baby toe and its neighbor.

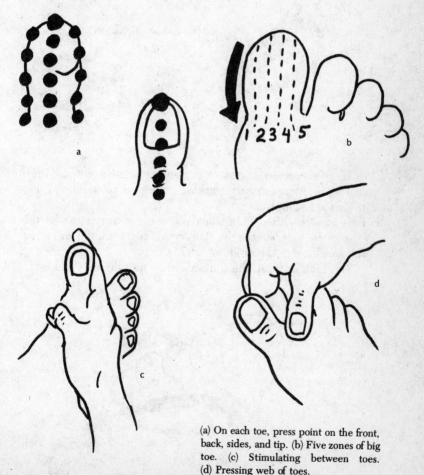

(a) On each toe, press point on the front, back, sides, and tip. (b) Five zones of big toe. (c) Stimulating between toes. (d) Pressing web of toes.

7. **Nail-inching.** On the skin that borders the sides and top only of the toenails, press and inch with your fingernail every eighth of an inch, using five to ten pounds pressure. Watch your patient's face to be sure you are not hurting. Then with your nail under his, gently flick each toenail upward away from toe. The nail of the thumb you press regular reflexes with should be short. The other thumbnail can be left slightly long and used for nail-inching.

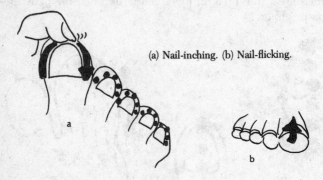

(a) Nail-inching. (b) Nail-flicking.

The nails receive and store electromagnetic current. By stimulating the periphery and flicking, energy is released and meridians are stimulated.

8. **Base stretch.** After stimulating the eye and ear points at the base of the toes, stretch the skin on this area from the far side of the small toe to the inside of the big toe.

This motion drains the sinuses and soothes the eyes and ears.

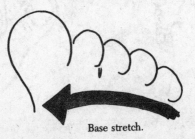

Base stretch.

9. *Toe effleurage.* Rub each toe from its tip down to its base to stimulate venous drainage.

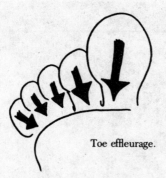

Toe effleurage.

STEP 5: SPECIFICS

1. *Points on the sole of the foot.* Working with Chart I, stimulate all the points on the foot. It is best to start on the spinal points first since all the body nerves branch out from them; work the spine from the sacral and lumbar area by the heel up to the cervical area by the big toe. Then work from the top of the foot down to the heel. Follow with friction and effleurage.

2. *Points for the lateral (outside) foot.* Press each point from the bottom of the heel up (see Chart II). Then rub (friction) the side of the foot with your knuckles, starting from the little toe all the way up to the ankle. Then rub up the outside of the Achilles tendon. Continue with effleurage.

   This side of the tendon stimulates the sacrum, lower back, and genitals.

3. *Points for the medial (inside) foot.* Press all points, giving special attention to kidney points (all around the ankle) and the fifth lumbar point. Friction with knuckle; then finish with effleurage.

4. *Points on the top of the foot.* Starting at the base of the toes, work the points shown on Chart II up to the leg-ankle junction. With your knuckles do friction over the entire top of foot, going from base of toes to the leg-ankle junction. Complete with effleurage.

5. *Points on the leg.*

a. *Friction.* Stimulate by using a wringing motion all the way up the leg to the knee.

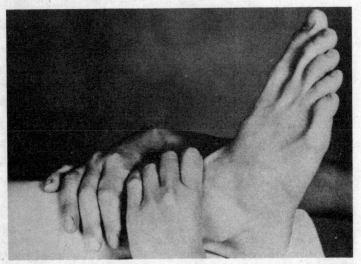

Friction on the leg, done up to the knee.

b. *Inside shin points.* Push your second, third, and fourth fingers under the shin bone (tibia). Do this all the way from top of the ankle to the knee bone.

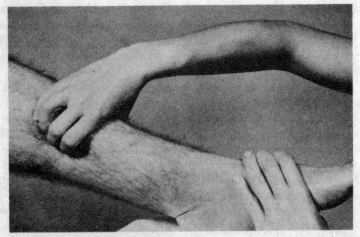

Stimulating inside shin points.

An especially important point for women along this vertical area is measured by the patient's fingers. It is the width of four fingers away from the ankle bone starting with the first finger placed in the center of the inside ankle. Known as the *menstrual point*, this point relieves cramps very rapidly and is good for other female disorders. Press in and hook under the shin bone at this point. Use as much pressure as the patient can tolerate. Hold until cramps subside.

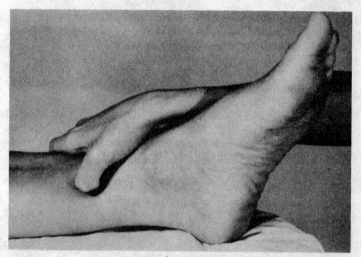

"Menstrual point," four fingers from middle of ankle.

Be on the lookout for swelling, granular tissue, and deposits in the shin area. Work them out by rubbing and sustained pressure. Such are common with women who experience congestion and tension in the genitals, especially when on the pill or using an IUD. Men with prostate trouble, tension, or degenerative tissue also have this symptom.

c. *Stomach 36 and lateral calf points*. Place the patient's hand on top of his knee and bend the knee slightly. Note where the middle finger falls in the groove between the tibia and fibula. This is Stomach 36, an important point for rejuvenating the entire system. Press this point with your thumb, while the middle finger of your other hand presses along the lateral (outside) calf points. Touch both points at the same time, but each is pressed deeply alternately. Stimulate Stomach 36 by pressing deeply and rubbing back and forth; then hold it lightly while you do deep rubbing on the lateral point. The thumb remains on the Stomach point while the other hand stimulates each lateral point starting from the top near the knee and going down toward the foot. Hold each point for five to ten seconds. Give sore spots and deposits extra attention. These points tonify the entire system.

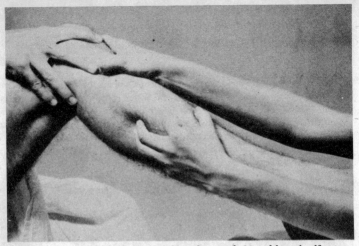

Alternating stimulation of Stomach 36 and lateral calf points.

d. *Center calf points.* Hold the leg with your left hand. Then your middle finger or knuckle presses up the center of the calf from the Achilles tendon to the soft indentation behind the knee, stimulating all the center calf points shown in Chart III.

This greatly stimulates endocrine glands, the adrenals especially. Watch the pressure; some highly stressed patients are very tender here.

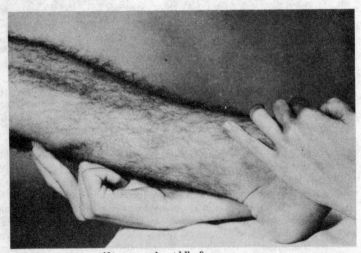

Stimulating center calf points with middle finger.

6. ***General Lymphatics movement.*** Placing one hand on top of leg at the ankle, push firmly all the way up to the top of the thigh. As soon as this one hand finishes, be doing the same with the other. Thus, there is a rapid, alternating, and constant push upward on the leg.

   The lymphatic drainage of the body depends on the pressure gradient in the body. As you push on the legs toward the heart, you increase the pressure in the body's periphery. This increases the flow of lymph as well as blood.

STEP 6: CLOSING

1. ***Tapotement.*** Clap your hands very firmly together, as if applauding, with loose wrists, but catch the foot, ankle, and calf in between your hands as you do so. ("Applauding" the feet!) You may also slap briskly or cup your palms and smack the calves. Or do it the butterfly way by slapping the foot at an angle and allowing your hands to brush a few inches of skin in an up and down motion.

Clapping tapotement.   Butterfly tapotement.

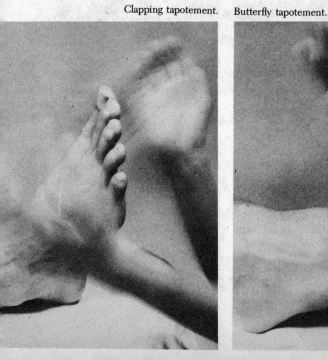
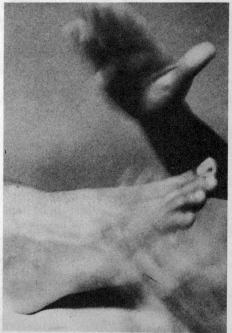

2. **Venous pump.** A very important part of the massage to stimulate the venous drainage to carry away the toxins. Begin at heel.
With thumb and forefinger stretch the Achilles tendon upward.
Now make a fist, and with your knuckles rub the calf very
firmly from the top of the tendon to the back of the knee. The
stroke should be upward and firm. If the leg has a lot of hair,
press your knuckles in and upward every few inches in a pumping manner. Repeat at least three times.

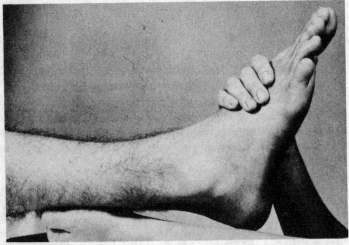

Venous pump.

The venous pump is stimulating the soleus muscle, deep in
the calf muscle, to increase venous drainage. The soleus contains most of the veins in the lower leg. Veins have no intrinsic
pumping system but are stimulated to pump toxins in the blood
by contracting movements of the muscle and respiration back
toward the heart and then on to the liver and kidneys for discharge. As you do this, have the patient take a few breaths and
exhale very deeply.

3. **Final effleurage.** Previously described as *Beginning effleurage.*
4. **Nerve stroke.** Rub your hands briskly to stimulate energy
centers in the middle of the palms. When they are warm, rapidly and gently brush the top of the skin so you barely touch the
hairs, from the knee, down the leg, and over the foot and toes.
Repeat at least three times.

5. *Final cleansing*. Repeat the nerve stroke but do it a few inches away from the skin to discharge any electromagnetic build-up from the body.

Optional. Before going on to the left foot, pause a moment with hands still gently on top of both feet. Have the patient become aware of the different feelings between the right and left foot. Then suggest to him or her to tune into the areas on the right side of the body that were previously blocked but now feel open and clear. Have him or her then try to experience, by contrast, the areas on the left side of the body that are still blocked, congested, and tense. Becoming aware of blockages is the first step toward letting them go.

STEP 7: REPEAT THE ABOVE SIX STEPS ON THE LEFT FOOT.

STEP 8: HEALING AFFIRMATION.

Every treatment should end with an affirmation. Place your palms gently on the top of the feet with your thumbs resting underneath the big toes. Project an image of the patient being well, whole, and with shining happiness. See him or her healed. See him or her in detail: hair, clothes, and expression. Hold the image for a few moments; then let go. And finally mentally state an affirmation. I usually say:

I affirm that healing is taking place. I am grateful for this opportunity to serve. The patient is healed.

It is possible for the practitioner to pick up negative vibrations and pain from the patient. This need not happen if you surround yourself with a visualization of white light and mentally affirm at the beginning and end of each treatment that you will not. After washing your hands under cold running water at the end of the treatment until the fingers feel cold, do some rapid nerve strokes down your own arms, fling your hands as if getting rid of something stuck to them, and affirm that you have not picked up any negative energy.

The Abbreviated Treatment

It is possible to abbreviate the Integrated Treatment to about fifteen minutes. While it is highly beneficial to the entire system, it is not so diagnostic, detailed, or specifically therapeutic. It concentrates on stimulating all the reflex points rather than on specific areas and on locating tender spots.

The outline is as follows:

STEP 1: OPENING

1. Patient does three deep breaths.
2. As he exhales, instruct him to make a mental command to "Relax!"
3. While he does this, you press both solar plexus points.

STEP 2: GENERAL MOVEMENTS

1. Beginning effleurage
2. Wringing stroke

STEP 3: ANKLE MOVEMENTS

1. Flexion, extension, and/or rotation
2. Plexus pull (optional)
3. Ankle points

STEP 4: TOE STROKES

1. Rotation
2. Toe pull with tendon stretch
3. Reflex points
4. Effleurage

STEP 5: SPECIFICS

1. *Points on the sole.* Divide the foot mentally into five parallel zones corresponding with the five toes. Stimulate all the points from the base of the toes to the heel, one zone at a time. If a tender spot comes to your attention, press for fifteen to twenty

seconds. But primarily you should be inching your thumb firmly and rapidly down each zone. Next do the same on the foot again but divide the sole into horizontal zones. You may wish to use both thumbs alternating pressure from each one as you proceed.

2. **Points for the lateral (outside) foot.** Again, divide the outside of the foot into zones and inch your thumb along. Give special attention to the genital point. This point is found by making an imaginary line from the center of the ankle to the farthest part of the heel. Bisecting this line is the area of the point. The box in the illustration signifies the general genital region. As you work this, press the exact opposite point on the inside ankle with the forefinger. This movement releases a lot of tension in the genital area and is very powerful.

3. **Points for the medial (inside) foot.** Divide into zones and inch. Give special attention to lower back point and genital point.

4. **Points on the top of the foot.** Stretch between the tendons from the base of the toes to the leg-ankle joint. Stimulate the lymphatics. Use knuckle friction and effleurage.

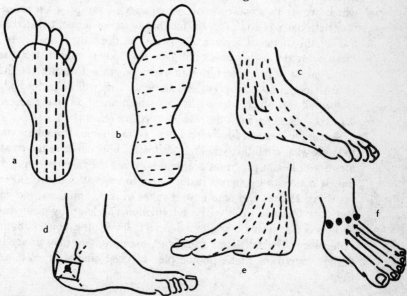

Zones for inching for Abbreviated Treatment.
(a) Vertical zones. (b) Horizontal zones. (c) Outside ankle. (d) Genital point. (e) Inside ankle. (f) Top of foot.

5. *Points on the leg.* Work inside shin points. Stomach 36 should be done alternately with center calf points.
6. *General Lymphatics.*

STEP 6: CLOSING

1. Tapotement
2. Venous pump
3. Final effleurage
4. Nerve stroke

STEP 8: REPEAT THE ABOVE ON LEFT FOOT.

STEP 9: HEALING AFFIRMATION

During the basic or abbreviated treatment, observe and remember the most troublesome (tender and granular) areas. Note to which organs these correspond. Then suggest the program or appropriate parts of the program for that organ or ailment, listed in the common ailment section. Focus first on the most tender areas, these being the body's weakest organ. The body is only as strong as the weakest organ. Start the therapy program focusing on the weakest organ or most prevalent ailment. This will help the body restore all the other minor ailments which are most likely secondary complications from the weakest organ's effect.

Keeping a record of each treatment is invaluable. It enables you to know what condition you first dealt with, how effective the treatments and health programs are, and how fast the body is responding. It makes the patient's history easy to read at a glance. Keep your own as well and note how changes in diet, emotions, etc. affect your feet and health. The information you learn by observing and recording can be of great help in developing your skills in reflexology. The following chart is an example; you may prefer to design your own. Make photocopies to keep charts for each patient.

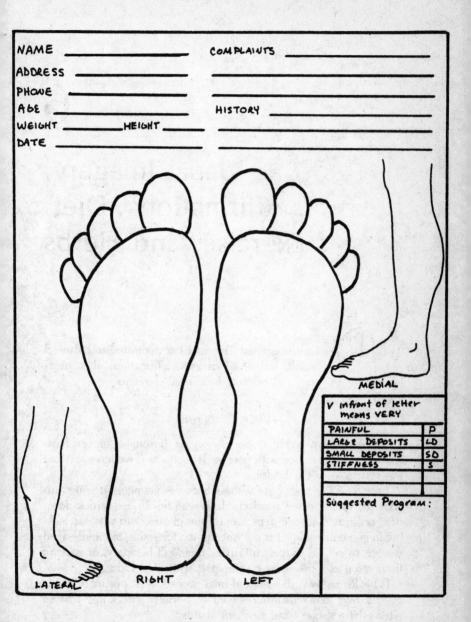

NAME _____

ADDRESS _____

PHONE _____

AGE _____

WEIGHT _____ HEIGHT _____

DATE _____

COMPLAINTS _____

_____

_____

HISTORY _____

_____

MEDIAL

V infront of letter means VERY	
PAINFUL	P
LARGE DEPOSITS	LD
SMALL DEPOSITS	SD
STIFFNESS	S

Suggested Program:

LATERAL   RIGHT   LEFT

6

Visual Imagery, Affirmations, Diet, Exercise, and Herbs

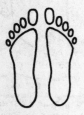 The Integrated Treatment is dedicated to balanced health, and visual imagery, affirmations, diet, exercise, and herbs are essential elements.

Visual Imagery

Healing today is big business—bigger hospitals, bigger bills, waiting rooms jammed with people. It seems as if we have less and less control over our health.

Each year the age of the victims becomes younger. It is not uncommon today to see small children who have been struck down with arthritis, who are dependent upon glasses, and who are lacking in good nutrition. It is not uncommon for young to middle-aged women to get rid of their uteruses, their gall bladders, or parts of their colon as if this were routine preparation for old age.

Is health really such a hit-and-miss process as it appears to be? Is control over one's health reduced to periodic check-ups that so often advise surgery and mechanical aids?

The answer is a resounding "No!"

Natural healing recognizes man's *own* ability to be healthy enough to resist disease or weak enough to be a receptive host for it.

Bugs attack plants that are raised in weak, unbalanced soil. Hardy plants resist attack. It is the same with all types of life. Our life style, diet, attitudes, and habits influence our resistance. It is a lowered resistance to disease that leaves us susceptible to disease—not the germs or the disease itself.

You have it within your reach to guarantee your own health by eliminating those things that cause weakened resistance. You can control many of the factors that control your health. The greatest influence in this is your mind. The physical body is never sick first; it is always the mind.

In some modern clinics where this has been recognized, for instance that of Dr. Irving Oyle in California, the first question a patient is asked is, "Why did you allow yourself to become ill?"

In his book *The Healing Mind* Dr. Oyle, a courageous and respected twentieth-century medical doctor, states:

This autonomous healing factor is under complete control of the psyche which by varying its rate of vibration can cause disease or initiate healing. . . . The role of the psyche as a cause of disease or as a medium of healing is something which each individual can test out in his own living experience. . . . It seems reasonable to assume that if we can get physiologically sick from responding psychologically to stress in some inappropriate way, we can perhaps get well by learning to control the physiologic response.

Oyle continued in his book:

I am suggesting the possibility that we humans may regain control over the behavior of our own bodies. Physicians throughout history, such as the sixteenth-century Paracelsus and the twentieth-century Carl Jung, have been attracted to the study of mental imagery as the quintessence of all healing rituals.

Many respected groups today are investigating "crystallized thought" or how our mind manifests in our bodies. It is not a fluke that such institutes as the American Institute for Noetic Sciences, headed by the former astronaut Edgar Mitchell, are researching this area. Nor is it strange that Dr. Carlton Simmonton, past director of the American Cancer Society, asks his cancer patients to visualize mentally the destruction of their own cancer cells.

We call this visual imagery, the process of using your imagination to see in your "mind's eye" a better state of health for yourself. This state then becomes manifest in your body. When mentally visualizing a healing image, your human consciousness initiates vibrations in the body and also in another postulated level of matter surrounding it, known as the bioplasma.

As a working tool, visual imagery accomplishes two important tasks:

1. It influences and heals the body.
2. It also treats the psyche; for unless the psyche is also treated, ill health will reappear in the same or a different form.

We are, then, the creators of our own physical reality. We can exude health and peace, or disease and disharmony. And we can visualize images of healing in a routine, guided program and conquer our physical manifestations of disease. It is time to let go of old prejudices and open up our minds, time to abandon "absolute" health programs that bring but feeble relief, and time to embrace, explore, and inaugurate methods that work. Visual imagery works. It is not dangerous and may be done anywhere by anyone. We can create our own health.

HOW TO PRACTICE VISUAL IMAGERY

Visual imagery requires a relaxed body and peaceful surroundings: any tension at all works against its effectiveness.

So, first, do some breath strokes (see chapter on strokes) to relax. Then visualize clearly the results you desire. Do this with closed eyes, and mentally focus and project your thoughts onto your forehead, just as if your thoughts were colorful images projected onto the blank screen of your mind (forehead). For example, if you have an infected finger, visualize, at your forehead, an image of the finger whole and healed. Hold the visual image for five to ten minutes, always bringing it back when it attempts to wander. Finish by stating an affirmation. Examples: "My finger is healed." "My stomach is relaxing." "My lungs are decongesting." Affirmation stamps the image onto your psyche and sets up a perfect stage for nature's healing forces to take over. Then let go, detaching yourself from the image and affirmation, stretch a bit, a couple more deep breaths, and go on your way.

In short then: deep breathe, visualize and hold the image, and then affirm the image.

Visual imagery should be practiced alone in a quiet place two to three times a day for as long as necessary. With constant practice, skill is acquired, and it then becomes possible to practice it anywhere, even when walking or jogging, although it is less distracting and more conducive to practice it in the same place at the same times each day. Be creative, too. Dr. Simmonton urges his cancer patients to visualize white blood cells as good-guy cowboys on white horses, galloping off to attack and conquer the bad cancer cells. He also stresses the importance of regular, daily sessions.

Visual imagery may be used by you to influence the health of others—even those not present. Mentally repeat that person's name, visualize what is wanted, and affirm it.

This is, then, one of the most important tools for practitioners to use in connection with the Integrated Treatment. Guided visualization exercises are offered in the appendix at the end of this chapter.

Diet

The whole matter of diet can easily get out of hand until it becomes alarming, confusing, and frequently a source of guilt. This is unfortunate and unnecessary.

The important thing about diet is to improve it to the degree that it is comfortable for you and contributes to your total balance.

Diet should bring harmony into one's life. For some people this will mean being a vegetarian; for others this will mean eating less red meats, more fish, and making sure to eat more vegetables and fruits.

So, diet is a personal thing. But even so, one can clean up one's act, improve one's menu, and make wise decisions about diet.

It is good, therefore, to have some general guidelines that remind us what to watch for.

Some nutritionists say we *must* have so many amino acids at one meal or exactly this many milligrams of this and that vitamin each day; one would have to keep constant score cards and tally up each mouthful. It all becomes too confusing to understand or remember, and it is unnecessary.

But if we break diet up into more general, manageable units, we can easily remember to: eat at least a half-dozen different vegetables a day, a few different fruits, at least one protein and one type of starch. The worry should not be complete protein but complete foods. The majority of your diet should be made up of complete, whole foods that are just as they came from nature, and are not missing essential elements due to refining processes. If you remember to eat whole vegetables, fruits, grains, seeds, nuts, and milk-cultured products, you'll get plenty of whole protein. Sprouts, legumes and grains that have been moistened and allowed to grow a few inches, are a live, vital food. If you eat meat, then remember to eat less red, fatty meat and more organ meats, fowl, fish, fresh eggs, soft, not hard, cheeses, plus the above mentioned foods; then you remember well.

I have my own preferences for food, like any other person. But I want to stress this fact: the whole thing about diet, important as it is, should not get out of hand and become an obsession. I mean this in both cases—the extreme indulgent and the extreme health nut. Ultimately, it is what comes from you that makes up who you are. And in the end, I think that "who you are" is what this life is all about, and how you use and serve your "youness" up to others.

DEVAKI'S TWO LAWS OF DIET

1. *Listen to feedback.* This is the whole trick of diet. How do you feel? Try new and different diets, give them enough time to enable you to judge the results, and then see how you feel. How do you look? How do your nails grow? How do your bowels move? How do you sleep? How do you interact with people?

In other words, are you eating that which contributes to your uplift of body and spirit? You and only you know the answer. So listen well to yourself.

2. *It's not what you do once in a while that matters, but what you do most of the time that really counts.* This means that you are searching for a consistent, balanced, and whole diet. You may go off it once in a while, but you should keep a consistent good habit. Then your foundations will not be shaken by an occasional ice-cream cone or a sociable dinner.

Observe also how the diet of another affects him or her. Does it, or does it not, inspire you to try it?

I eat a vegetarian diet and many raw foods. But I cannot promise how I will eat tomorrow. I remain flexible; and if tomorrow that voice inside calls for an egg, or a piece of fish, I will eat an egg or a piece of fish. But I will eat with love and a bowl of sprouts! If our goal is awareness, we should keep ourselves spontaneous and open. We should not be afraid to try vegetarianism, and not afraid to give it up, not be afraid to fast, and not afraid to eat. "Life" is what diet is all about.

RULES FOR ANY DIET

1. Systematically under-eat. (The worst curse is a tongue out of control!)
2. Take a few moments before and after each meal to:

   - Enjoy a few deep breaths.
   - Bless the food and make an affirmation to raise it to its highest perfection.
   - Give thanks for having some fuel in front of you.

3. Chew thoroughly.
4. Eat when you eat. Give yourself up to eating—not to T.V., the morning paper, and other activities that distract from the thoroughness of your chewing and compete for the available blood.
5. If you have discomfort after a meal, skip the next one.

GUIDELINES FOR THE SANE DIET

The Sane Diet consists of two parts: five personal variables depending on your life style and four general guidelines that, when combined with the five personal variables, bring satisfaction, fulfillment, and a balanced diet.

Five Personal Variables. Your diet should be planned with respect to:

1. *How physically and mentally active you are.* Increased physical activity can handle more calories and heavier foods, but don't kid yourself. Increased mental activity is heightened through less calories.
2. *The weather.* Cold weather allows the body to handle some heavier foods; the opposite holds true in warm weather.
3. *Locality.* It is best to have a large part of your diet consist of foods that thrive within your geographic area.
4. *Your attitude.* How you feel matters as much as what you eat. Meal times should be pleasant, serene, or jovial. (It is not the time to tell your family you're fed up and leaving tomorrow for Capistrano.)
5. *Your personal fire* (your ability to digest and assimilate the food). It is not how much you eat but how much you assimilate that counts. Eat only what your stomach can handle.

Four General Guidelines.

1. *Eat a colorful meal.* Each color has specific mineral and vitamin values: red, black, and blue means iron; green means magnesium; orange and yellow means vitamin A. Foods when in season are at their highest value in color and nutrients.
2. *Eat a varied diet daily.* Four to six different vegetables a day, and most important, eat at least three which grow above ground; at least one piece of fruit but preferably two; protein; few starches (two for the kids but one for adults); and plenty of fruit and vegetable juices and water but not at the same time you are eating solids.
3. *Eat a diet that maintains a proper acid-alkaline balance.* This means about 80 per cent alkaline and 20 per cent acid (see chart in chapter appendix).
4. *At least half your daily diet should be raw.* As many fruits, vegetables, sprouts, nuts, and seeds as possible should be eaten raw. But when cooking, steam, bake, or broil whenever possible,

using the remaining liquids to drink. Avoid salt, which draws out nutrients and moisture. Avoid fried and fatty foods. Also avoid cooking more vegetables than you will use immediately, for when refrigerated they lose much of their value.

SOME USEFUL DOS AND DON'TS ON DIET

- Eat your vegetables and fruits at separate meals.
- Eat concentrated proteins and concentrated starches at separate meals (see food list in chapter appendix).
- Avoid eating carbohydrates with acid foods.
- Avoid eating concentrated starches with concentrated sugars (winter squash with honey, for instance).
- Eat melons by themsleves, not with other fruits.
- Drink milk separate from your meals if you have any trouble whatsoever with digestion.

Remember, it is how you eat most of the time that counts. Don't be afraid of discipline. Although you should clean up your diet at a rate that is comfortable for you, you should not be afraid when necessary to tell yourself "No"; too much indulgence in flexibility accomplishes little. But neither should you go to the opposite extreme. If you deprive yourself of something too long, your ego gets back by wanting even more of it later. And be gentle in all your diet transitions. Moderation and gentle persistence are always the best approach to diet, and to life.

THE PLAGUE: OVEREATING

Have you been vaccinated against the disease of overeating? *The serum: will power.*

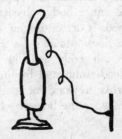

This is a mouth.

This is a vacuum cleaner.

They are different. But most people think they are the same. People think they can suck down food and that it will then be automatically churned and taken care of by magic grinders and waste bags, somewhere down below the neck. They will then complain about their doctor bills. Yet they think nothing of eating at Ulcer Gulch restaurants, and paying a pretty penny for the privilege of overeating and doing their health in.

Of course, we all become attached to food. It's the easiest form of satisfaction that one can obtain alone.

But no matter how much exercise you get, how organic and healthy a diet you eat, or how spiritually you behave, overeating has the power to cancel out a lot of angels.

A holy man once said, "No matter how many prayers, masses or temples you attend, if you overeat, all you get is food." You get more than that. You get trouble. Even if one doesn't drink alcohol, overeating produces it, as a toxic ferment in the body together with poisonous gases, pressure against all the organs, and constant blood depletion from the brain and other organs. It does no one any good.

I will even go so far as to say it is better to eat a poorer diet in sparse moderation, than a gluttonish gorge of organic goodies.

My favorite definition of a holy man is one who has complete control over all nine holes in his body. One can do this only if one isn't selfish and has complete trust and respect for this body as a gift from the Creator.

Exercise

Exercise is equally as important as visualizations and diet. Just as visualizations nourish the body emotionally and psychically, and as diet feeds and maintains the physical body, exercise contributes energy to the entire body, physically, mentally, and psychically. Exercise is food. It draws oxygen, one of our most powerful foods and cleansers, deep into all cells. The more we exercise, the more blood vessels our body actually grows, to accommodate more nourishing blood stimulated by the activity. As you exercise, use the breath stroke to work out tension, stiffness, to give you more energy and enhance the benefits of the exercise.

All good health starts with a healthy bloodstream, needed to feed and build healthy cells. This comes from a good diet. All good health depends on the blood circulating quickly enough to reach all the cells. This is greatly influenced by exercise.

And all good health depends on rest. This depends on attitude and discipline. As you visualize, relax and let go of worry. Rest cures. Rest rebuilds energy and restores balance. Discipline yourself to take time to rest, to visualize positive progress, and to relax yourself into excellent health.

Herbs

Herbs are used in this book because they are natural, effective, and easy to use. The use of plants is nature's oldest form of medicinal healing. Herbs, as mentioned in this book, can be used as either a tea or powdered and taken in gelatin capsules, two with each meal.

The tea is made by placing a heaping teaspoonful of herb per cup of boiling water, removing pot from the fire, and allowing the mixture to steep for twenty minutes. The water should not be chlorinated or flouridated if possible. Distilled water is the best. The water should ideally be boiled in non-metallic utensils, and never in aluminum pots. The herbs should never be boiled, although root herbs should be allowed to simmer for twenty minutes, not steep.

Herbs used for medicinal purposes when taken as a tea should be taken three times a day, one or two cups at a time, in between meals. Ideally, they should not be taken with any kind of sweetener, including honey.

Appendix to Chapter

GUIDED VISUALIZATION EXERCISES

- Do not eat one hour before or one half hour after exercises.
- Prepare yourself with the breath stroke.
- Mentally focus all visualization at your forehead, with eyes closed.
- End each exercise with an affirmation.

Triangle Visualization. Visualize a triangle of any size. Once you "see" this, visualize an object in the lower right-hand corner that symbolizes you, the way you are now. Then in the left-hand corner, see an object that symbolizes how you would like to be. Ask: "Self, what is preventing me from being this?" Let the answer come as an object at the top of the triangle. Think about what appears, and what meaning it can have for you.

Four-Part Visualization. (Dr. Carl Jung believed that an equal-armed cross and the concept of 4 were images that could initiate healing.) Visualize a circle divided into four parts by an equal-armed cross. In Space 1 (upper right-hand corner), see an image of yourself as you look today. In Space 2 (lower right-hand corner) focus in on a personal problem, and how it looks to you. If you have a tumor, you may see a wrinkled mass or a black circle. In Space 3 (lower left-hand corner) visualize yourself doing things to help this problem. Let the images appear spontaneously. In Space 4 see yourself in your most perfect vision of yourself. Affirm: "I am becoming this; I am healed."

Reaching-Up Visualization. (This gets rid of depression and tiredness in minutes.) Sit erect with both arms above your head. Reach alternately with your hands toward the ceiling. Visualize your hands grabbing vitality and energy. See it flow down your arms and settle on your neck, shoulders, and chest. When you feel re-energized and refreshed, stop.

Visualization Bath. Add ¼ cup apple cider vinegar and ⅓ cup Clorox bleach (do not use any other bleach!) to a hot tub. Soak for twenty minutes. First ten minutes, do slow deep breathing. Visualize life, vitality, and peace filling you up with each inhale so that you become more and more buoyant, and visualize any problem leaving with the exhale. Relax ten more minutes.

Affirmations to commit to memory, to be said at any time, especially at the end of visualization exercises.

1. Everyday, in everyway, I am getting better and better.
2. "I sought the Lord, and He heard me, and delivered me from all my fears." Psalm 34:4.
3. I lean on my faith and am healed.

ACID AND ALKALINE FOODS

Digestion of foods leaves an ash in the body. These ashes are alkaline or acid. The body requires about 80 per cent alkaline foods and 20 per cent acid foods.

High Alkali-Forming Foods

Figs
Soy and lima beans
Apricots
Spinach, turnip, and beet greens
Raisins and dates
Almonds
Carrots
Cucumbers
Cantaloupe
Greens (e.g., lettuce, parsley, collards, etc.)
Potatoes

High Acid-Forming Foods

Fish (oysters are highest)
Veal
Organ meats
Most meat and fowls
Eggs
Grains (except millet, buckwheat, or when sprouted)
Nuts (except almonds or brazil)

CLASSIFICATION OF FOODS

Proteins

Nuts (most)
All cereals
Dry beans and peas
Soybeans
Flesh foods (not fat)
Milk products
Olives
(Avocados, comfrey, and brussel sprouts have surprisingly large amounts of protein.)
Peanuts

Fat

All oils
Butter
Cream
Nuts
Avocados
Fat meats
Lard

Acid Fruits

Citrus fruits
Pineapple
Pomegranates
Tomatoes
Sour grapes, peaches, plums, apples

Sub-Acid Fruits

Fresh figs
Pear
Sweet peach, apple,
  cherry, plum
Papaya
Apricot
Mango
Cherimoya
Berries

Sweet Fruits

All dried fruits
Bananas
Dates, breadfruit, carob
Thomson and muscat
  grapes
Prunes
Ripe persimmon

Starches

All cereals
Dry beans (not soy) and
  peas
Potatoes
Chestnuts and peanuts
Hubbard and banana
  squash
Pumpkin
Jerusalem artichoke
Caladium root

Mildly Starchy

Carrots
Rutabaga
Parsnip
Cooked turnip
Salsify

Non-Starchy Green Vegetable Succulents

All succulent vegetables
without regard to
color.

Melons

Watermelon	Pie melon
Musk	Persian
Casaba	Banana melon
Crenshaw	Nutmeg
Cantaloupe	Honeydew
Christmas	Honey balls

Special Programs

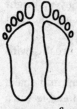

The Integrated Treatment may be used in any situation. However, it is felt that shortened reflexology treatments, combined with balanced health programs for specific situations, fulfill a definite need.

When using the special programs, follow each one carefully. Each reflexology treatment, unless otherwise specified, should be done for five minutes, morning and night. Have patience; nature works steadily and slowly, but *thoroughly.*

Morning Wake-Up

How you wake up is very important. It affects your whole day. You can influence the way you arise, and the energy you receive from it.

Waking up is a transition. It is a time of getting up and being active after lying on your back in a subconscious non-physically active state for many hours. It is therefore important that you respect this transition, and make rising as gentle as possible. Getting up too quickly from sleep is a special affront to the glands, which control your youth, beauty, and vitality.

Here is a guided outline for waking up that takes five to ten minutes, does not shock the system or glands, and rejuvenates the whole body.

- Upon first awakening, train yourself to make a positive affirmation automatically. An example: "I am full of life and vitality. I will have a great day."
- Stretch from side to side, while still in bed, and then stretch lengthwise with arms above your head. This begins to circulate the blood throughout the body and rebalances your energies.
- Rapidly and firmly massage yourself all over. Just a few moments of this helps oxygenate the body and feed the cells.
- If the sun is shining or there is light in the room, open your eyes slowly, allowing a bit of light at a time to hit your eyes. Bright lights suddenly striking the eyes shock the entire nervous and glandular systems.
- Sit on the edge of your bed, and take three deep breaths with exaggerated exhales to clear the lungs of stale air.
- Still sitting on the edge, lean back, lift your feet up and shake and bang the soles together as fast and hard as possible for a count of ten.
- Press the points on each big toe (pineal, pituitary, brain), and rotate the toe three times in each direction. Press the tips of all toes.
- On one foot at a time do tapotement (clapping and slapping the entire foot and leg).
- Leave the bed and sit in the polarity squat for one minute to bring energy into the body and stimulate its circulation.

Polarity squat. Squat on feet placed flat on the ground. Sit with buttocks as close to ground as possible. You can remain steady in this posture, or sway from side to side, forward and backward, or in circles. The benefits of this squat are taught as part of Dr. Randolph Stone's Polarity Therapy.

- Stand up. Inhale as you stretch up on your toes and reach upward with your arms. Exhale fully as you bend over, head toward the floor. Hold the exhale for a count of eight. Then, still leaning over, rap your head, neck, and shoulders firmly with your knuckles for another count of eight. Inhale as you stretch up again. Repeat three times.
- Run cold water over your feet for at least one minute. Rub them dry briskly with a rough towel.
- Sit quietly for a minute. See a mental image of yourself in the happiest, healthiest, and handsomest way you can idealize. Project this image strongly onto your mind and make an affirmation, "I am this!"

- Do not listen to loud music or eat for at least half an hour. The body, like a machine, needs to warm up before properly serving you. Water or room-temperature liquid may be taken, but avoid coffee, commercial tea, and very hot drinks, which bombard and weaken the glands.

RECOMMENDED MORNING DRINKS

- Maté and peppermint tea, mixed together. This is stimulating, and without the negative traits of coffee or commercial tea.
- Pure grape juice with a dash of cayenne pepper, for energy.
- Raspberry leaf tea. This tastes much like commercial tea, and is healthful. It helps drain excess fluids and tones the body.
- A good morning wake-up for the thyroid: Squeeze the juice of one half grapefruit into a cup of warm water. Spoon the fleshy part of the fruit into the water, too. Drink slowly. This drink curbs appetite and activates metabolism.

RECOMMENDED BREAKFASTS

- Fresh fruit in proper combinations (see Some Useful Dos and Don'ts on Diet).
- Vegetable or fruit juice.
- Carrot juice blended with yeast, sprouts, and a dash of vanilla.
- Yogurt with 2 T. of ground seeds or nuts or raisins.
- Grain cereals. Try soaking them overnight and eating them raw the next morning. Or mix them with a little butter even when they are raw. A good combination is barley and millet with a little chia and poppy seed.
- Try skipping breakfast and wait until lunch. Your body cleanses at night; if you skip breakfast, it will continue to cleanse until about eleven o'clock.

MORNING SHOWER

To get all the good we should out of a shower, it should consist of:

- Skin brushing: Brush yourself all over, firmly, with a skin brush or loufa sponge. Nothing makes the skin so soft and pleasant to touch as daily skin brushing.
- A five to ten minute hot shower followed by ice cold; then both repeated. The long period of hot water stimulates the parasympathetic nervous system. The alternating of hot and cold water builds up your resistance and physical strength. Ending with cold closes the pores, so you have less chance of getting chilled, or being receptive to airborne germs.

EVENING SHOWER

After a hot shower, finish by rubbing the entire body with a mixture of ½ cup apple cider vinegar with ½ cup of peppermint tea. Then run the feet under cold water. Do a firm foot tapotement and finish with three nerve strokes.

REFLEXOLOGY WAKE-UP EXERCISE . . . THIS IS THE MOST IMPORTANT EXERCISE IN THIS BOOK!

When you are in a hurry, doing just the following exercise will energize and balance your whole body. It stimulates all the foot reflex points, circulates oxygen, and deepens the breath.

Step 1. Sit on your heels, take a deep inhalation, stretching up and back as you do so. Support your weight by pressing your

Reflexology Wake-Up Exercise, Step 1.

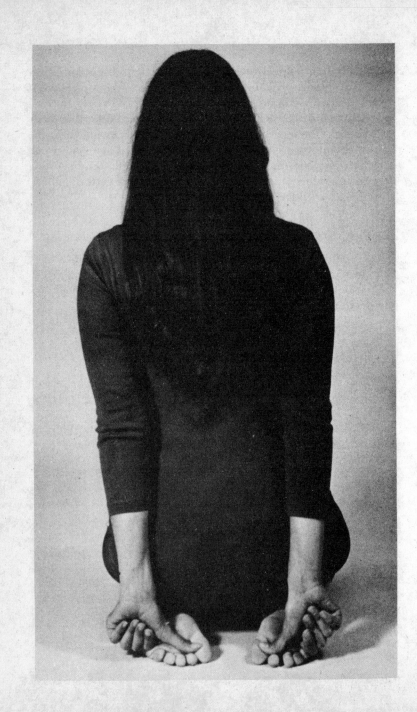

thumbs into your big toes, and your knuckles on the floor. Count to five. Lean back, expand your chest, push your shoulders back, and elongate your neck as much as possible. Optional: With each inhalation, mentally "affirm" a trait that you want to develop such as vitality or will power.

Step 2. Now exhale and bend as far forward as you can, the goal being touching the floor while keeping your buttocks on your heels. Rest your hands on the soles of your feet. Optional: With each exhalation, mentally affirm a trait you want to let go of. For example: "I let go of being angry."

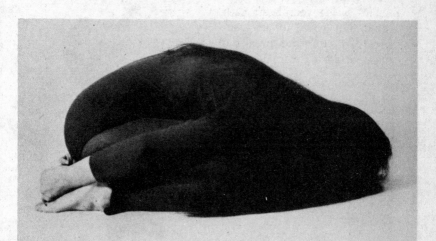

Reflexology Wake-Up Exercise, Step 2.

Step 3. Repeat the inhaling and stretching back, but press into the next toe to stimulate a new reflex. Do this for each toe. Then repeat the entire soles of your feet by using your knuckles.

Finally, sit up and remain silent for one minute. See an image of yourself that is radiant, full of energy, and happy.

Go and have a good day.

LIFE-CONQUERS-ALL EXERCISE

This is a wonderful morning exercise to seal yourself in positivity for the day, and give an internal massage to your organs. It consists of three parts:

Step 1. Stand up. Inhale slowly and completely while arching your spine up and backward. As you do this, swing your arms in circles with your palms facing your heart each time they come toward you. Feel that you are drawing all the positive attributes of life into your heart.

Life-Conquers-All Exercise, Step 1.

Step 2. Exhale loudly as you bend forward, head toward the ground. As you do so, repeat the circular movements with your hands, this time palms pushing away from you. Feel that you are getting rid of unwanted habits, tension, and disease.

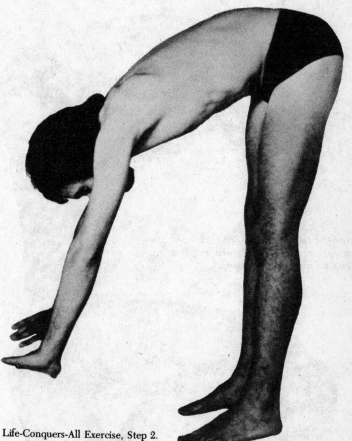

Life-Conquers-All Exercise, Step 2.

Step 3. Remain fully bent over. Place your hands on your knees, pressing slightly against them for support. Exhale fully, and pull your stomach as far back as possible, as though it could touch your spine. Then abruptly release your stomach. Repeat this pulling in and releasing, or flapping of your stomach, as long as you can comfortably hold your breath out. Inhale and rise up, repeating the exercise at least two more times.

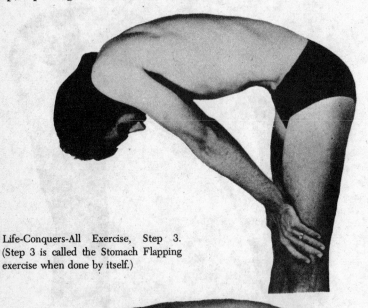

Life-Conquers-All Exercise, Step 3. (Step 3 is called the Stomach Flapping exercise when done by itself.)

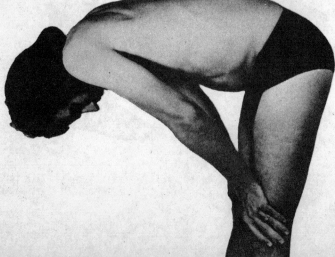

ROCKING ON THE SPINE

This is an excellent way to massage the entire spine, stimulate the flow of cerebro-spinal fluid, and energize your system.

- While on your back, hug your head to your knees.
- Inhale and rock backward as far as possible.
- Exhale and rock forward as far as possible.

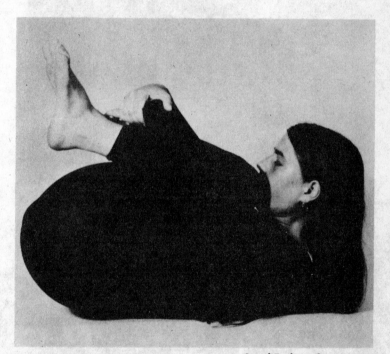

Spinal Rocking, first position.

- Continue at least ten times. If you do this for about one hundred times, it's equivalent to two Swedish massages, a chiropractic adjustment, and an "A" on a term paper. You may also try this alternative position: crossing your legs, holding your big toes, and rocking back and forth.

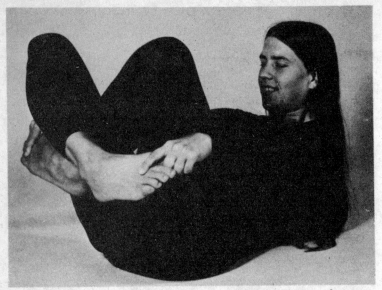

Spinal Rocking, second position.

Couples

If more people took the time to rub each other's feet, there would be more understanding and love, and less divorce.

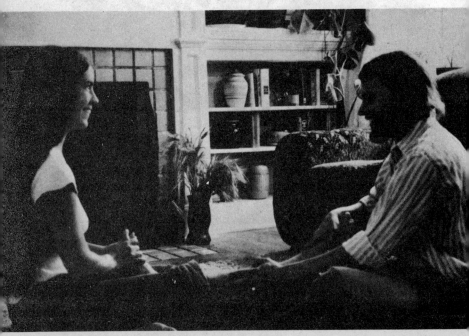

COUPLE'S WAKE-UP

Couples can give each other, and at the same time, themselves five-minute reflexology treatments while still in bed. While doing this, make an affirmation together, such as, "We are lucky to have each other. We are lucky to have another day. We will use it well."

After the polarity squat, get up and stretch. One person at a time should gently pound, with loose fists, the spine of the other. One stands, bent over, with head toward the floor, while the other percusses the spine and back from the buttocks to the head, including all the shoulders, neck, and scalp. Then trade off.

COUPLE'S EVENTIDE

After a long day, draw a warm scented bath. Both sit on the side of the tub. Each soaks one foot in the water while giving the other foot to the mate to share treatments. Concentrate on the big toes, spine, calves, and effleurage. Finish with a cup of tea or share a piece of fruit. This outline may be used after an argument, or better yet, during one.

FERTILITY PROBLEMS

If one has trouble becoming pregnant, here is a program that should be practiced by both:

- Abstain from sex for two weeks. This is a must.
- Reflexology: Each day, morning and night, for five minutes, stimulate the genital reflexes, spinal reflexes, adrenal glands, solar plexus, colon and pancreas, and all the points on the big toes. Make sure you always end with one solid minute of tapotement, venous pump fifteen times, and effleurage. Finish with a joint affirmation (which should also be affirmed upon arising and retiring). An example: "We are going to have a beautiful child."
- Diet: Eat a menu high in raw foods, especially whole grains, nuts, cabbage, fruit and leafy greens. Each day have at least 1 T. each of sunflower, sesame and pumpkin seeds. Take 250 mg of

Couple sharing Integrated Treatment.

chelated zinc, 400 I.U. of Vitamin E, and a balanced B-complex dose daily.

- Fast the day you will resume activities.
- First massage each other's feet, focusing on the points prescribed above. End with very firm affirmations.
- Use the visualization stroke. See energy going down through the tops of your heads, into your hearts and reproductive organs.
- Continue this regime until you have success. Have fun and have a baby.

EXERCISE FOR BOTH PARTNERS TO STRENGTHEN REPRODUCTIVE ORGANS

- Stand up, placing your hands on your knees. Take a deep breath, then exhale fully.
- On exhalation, lean over, and squeeze up your reproductive organs and anus as tightly as possible, as though holding back a bowel movement.
- Then fully release the muscles. It is squeezing and releasing these muscles and organs that stimulates their blood flow, nutrition, and tone. Repeat at least twenty-five times.
- Inhale as you stand up, relax, and do a healing visualization. Imagine the inner environment of your reproductive organs. "See" them well, functioning normally.

EXERCISE FOR PARTNERS

Place soles of feet so they are touching, hold hands, and lift feet up together. Keep mutual eye contact while breathing deeply

Couple's exercise.

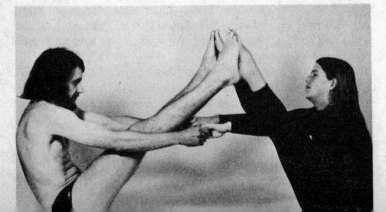

together for one to three minutes. This mutually stimulates each other's foot reflexes and creates a bond of shared energy.

Child-Care Situations: Babies

BABY'S FOOT TREATMENT

- Note well: Use a scented homemade cream if you do use one. Never use anything on your baby's skin that the baby could not eat, because the body absorbs whatever is put on the skin. Never use mineral oil; it robs the baby of vitamins. And never use commercial talcums, which usually have high metallic and asbestos counts and are toxic to the human system.
- You can do all the strokes of the basic or abbreviated Integrated Treatment except those that pull firmly or sharply, such as the plexus pull, nail-inching, or strong tapotement.
- *Be gentle!* Do not press too hard, especially on the toes; but still look for tender spots and hold them until they feel released. Sing or deep breathe while you press. Keep your vibrations relaxed and confident.
- Most babies enjoy having their feet in warm water. Try massaging underwater.
- Emphasize the spinal reflexes, toes, and lymphatics. When a baby is learning to crawl or walk, emphasize the foot, hip, spinal, sciatic nerve, and glandular reflexes.

NEWBORN'S TREATMENT

You can gently massage a newborn, right after birth, in a tub of room-temperature, clean (not city) water. Rub the body and feet very gently and slowly. No pulling or stretching, just gently stroking. Make no loud noises. Feel relaxed and joyous. Make an affirmation, "This child is a light, a blessing, a gift. This child is well, whole, and happy."

FOR ANXIOUS, CRABBY, COLICKY BABIES

- Alternate pressing the solar plexus on both feet, and then the coping reflex (see Chart I). Hold each for thirty seconds at a time.

- Then place one hand on the forehead, the other on the navel. Gently rock the hand on the navel, back and forth. Do not rub. Hold the hand in place, but rock it.

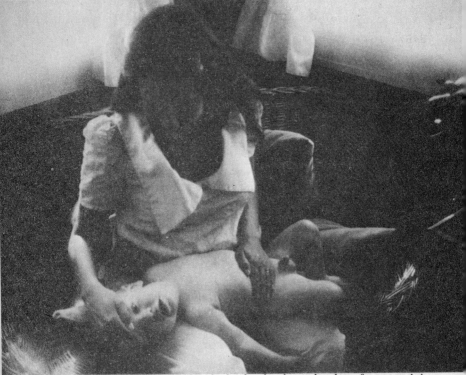

Holding forehead and rocking solar plexus for anxious baby.

- Keep one hand on the navel, rocking, while your other hand moves from the forehead to the solar plexus points on the feet and back to the forehead. Next the coping reflex. Continue alternating, holding each point for thirty seconds. Continue this for ten to fifteen minutes. As you rock, do some deep breathing yourself. As you mentally calm yourself while holding and rocking the child's navel, you will enhance the calming effect on the child.
- The child, once calm, may be given some dilute camomile or slippery elm tea with 1 tsp. of molasses.

EXERCISE FOR BABY BEFORE BABY WALKS

Hold your baby upside down so the head hangs comfortably and the arms reach a chair, the floor, or some solid surface. Once into a position the baby enjoys, let him explore this new vantage point. Babies learn to use their arm muscles and walk on their hands while you support them. After a few failures, repeats, and possibly a bit of mild fright, they come to like and enjoy it. This is good for circulation, arm muscles, brain, and future general health.

Baby exercise before he or she can walk. This is good to do even when they are walking to strengthen the arms.

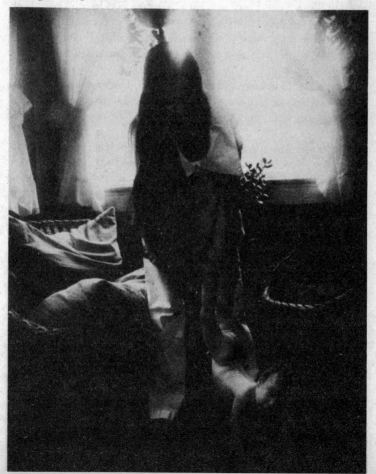

CHILD-CARE DIET

Your child's diet affects his entire life. You have to be really aware of this since most food companies try to gyp you. In scientific studies it has been documented that salt in baby foods creates a positive trend toward hypertension and high blood pressure in later life. Mother's milk has 0.4 gram sodium chloride per liter in contrast to cow's milk, which has three times the salt content. Salt in commercial formulas is equal to the proportion in cow's milk, which is intended for a small calf expected to gain several hundred pounds in its first year.

Babies' habits are formed by how you feed them early in life. Don't start them on salt, sugar, or starch habits. Breastfeeding early in life is a good way to insure that the child has the very best. If you can't breastfeed, try giving soy or seed milks with 1 tsp. molasses before you resort to cow's milk or formulas. If you use cow's milk, dilute one part milk to one part cardamom tea to help the child's digestion.

Do not start feeding solid foods too soon. Understand that babies are not equipped to eat solid foods, especially starches such as cereals and crackers, for at least six months! This cannot be stressed enough.

Starch digestion and some assimilation begins in the mouth. When we chew well, salivary amylase is mixed with starch to break it down. Since babies can't chew well with no teeth, the digestion is very incomplete. Starches then ferment in the intestinal tract, causing gas, congestion, and mucus. Generally, babies will react by being cranky, colicky, and becoming puffed in appearance and difficult or dull in temperament.

This is the reason that primitive, native mothers chewed the food in their own mouths first. The food began to break down because of the salivary amylase in their own mouths. Then they gave it to the child.

When a baby gets teeth and can chew fairly well, then nature is saying he is ready to eat starches.

Starches and solid foods served too early and too often in infancy are tickets for trouble later. It is no coincidence that younger and younger adults develop arthritis, hypoglycemia, cancer, genital weaknesses and illnesses. The gall bladder that has to be removed at age thirty-eight could have begun its trouble in constant irritation during infancy by undigested starches in the digestive tract. It is not normal to have stones and organs removed, or to live in fear of so many diseases. Old age was not meant to be so full of the hell that our life styles have produced.

Do not overfeed your baby. This cannot be emphasized strongly enough. Fat cells increase very rapidly during early childhood. Once formed, they never go away. They can easily pull fatty acids out of the bloodstream and swell up. It becomes a real effort to keep them "down." Thus fat children will have an extra hard time keeping off undesired weight as they grow older. Overfeeding stresses all organs and tissues and sets the stage for poor physical constitution, lack of resistance, and emotional problems, no matter how high a quality of food the fat is formed from.

FAMILY MASSAGE

It is good to get into the habit of the family working together on their health, making health consciousness a natural part of your child's world.

At night, sit the family in a circle. This can also be done with groups of friends. Each person takes the right foot of the person next to him. Give a mini-treatment to the foot. Then switch and do the left foot.

Family or group massage.

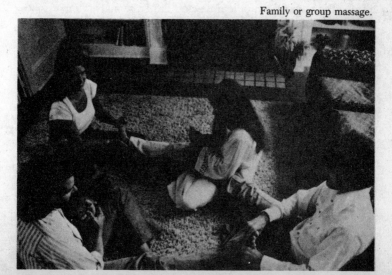

After this, it is nice for the family to share a cup of tea, and to brush and floss their teeth together. Finish with a family affirmation. (One of the parents might guide everyone through a visualization.)

When a child is sick, have the whole family give him a treatment. Have each member take a limb and work the basic strokes, or several effleurages. Use breath and visualization, too.

Child-Care Situations: Childhood Illnesses

The following are some frequent childhood illnesses. Remember that each of these is a symptom. Attend to the illness, but look for the causes in the child's life style, diet, exercise, and emotional and academic life.

EARACHES

Children often have earaches and spend nights and days in crying pain. I have seen this pain rapidly diminished by dipping a cotton ball in garlic juice (made by blending 1 clove of garlic with ¼ cup water in the blender) and placing it in the child's ear. Onions or warmed olive oil may be used as garlic substitute. If the child is subject to frequent earaches, mullein oil may be added to the garlic juice. After the ear is packed, rub the feet with another cotton ball dipped in the garlic juice, or with a raw clove. Then find the most tender ear points and hold them for one-minute intervals, alternating with fifteen effleurage and fifteen venous pump strokes. Finally take hold of the ear lobe firmly and rapidly pull it downward, forward, and up. Repeat this three times.

Earaches are often signs of faulty diet or digestion. The child should be placed on a juicy fruit diet until the earache subsides. When the child is better, keep the diet light. Give lots of fruits and vegetables, omitting heavy starches and proteins, especially dairy products and red meats, for several days to one week. Keep the ear packed with a cotton ball saturated with three drops of mullein oil. Change the pack three to four times a day.

Whenever a baby or child (or even an adult) shows signs of disturbing earaches, sore throats, or painful gas, administer an enema.

A child's enema is done by filling an ear syringe with lukewarm water. Oil the tip. Place tip gently into rectum and slowly squeeze liquid in. Hold your finger over the anal opening for fifteen seconds. Then release. Do this in a small tub. Repeat until water released is clear. Naturally, it is very important to consult your doctor *before* administering an enema to a child. Overuse of enemas for anyone is not desirable.

FEVERS

I feel that fever, unless very high, such as 104 degrees and above, is usually a good thing. It is nature's way of "burning" the toxins that are polluting the body, yes, even a young body. If fevers are not very high, they should be allowed to run their course, and the following procedures will help the body "burn" the toxins with less wear and tear on the tissues. However, if there seems to be any cause to worry, contact a physician at once and do not hesitate to use drugs or techniques the physician prescribes.

Reflexology for Fevers. Keep one hand on the forehead, the other free, and stimulate the sides of the toes and metatarsals. Give special attention to the cervical region on both big toes. Press both solar plexus reflexes and hold for one minute. Then press the fever point with a ball-point pen, the point hidden inside the pen. Do lymphatics and venous pump, fifteen times each. End by holding the coping reflexes on each foot simultaneously for one to five minutes.

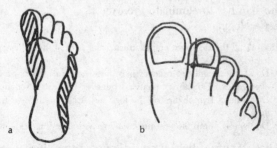

(a) Reflex areas for fevers. (b) Press point with ball-point pen, the nib retracted. Hold for thirty seconds. Release, rub, repeat two more times.

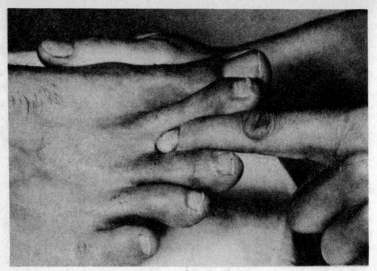

Coping point. Pressing indentation between second and third toes.

After the reflexology treatment, you may rub the feet with garlic, cinnamon, or clove oil. Cinnamon and clove oil, which are not so effective as garlic, may either be used separately or combined in a mixture with equal parts of each.

Do not feed solid food to a child with a fever. Dilute peppermint and cardomon tea are very soothing.

RASHES

Though a rash can indicate a variety of problems, it is often a sign that the body's organs of elimination are being overloaded so that the skin has to eliminate the excess.

Reflexology.

- Work all the digestive points, tracing the path of the colon by inching, at least five times.
- Do all the lymphatic reflexes five times each, all the big toe points and liver reflex. (Do the lymphatics whenever you can throughout the day.) Do General Lymphatics on the legs and arms, twenty-five times on each limb.
- Do venous pump fifteen times, ending with effleurage fifteen times.

Diet. During this time, do not serve heavy proteins or starches; instead keep to juicy fruits and raw and steamed vegetables as much as possible. A dilute tea of burdock root and comfrey helps cleanse and soothe the system.

Rash Lotion. Make *aloe vera* water: Lacerate the succulent inner leaves of the aloe vera cactus plant, the plant capable of effecting faster healing than any other plant in nature. Cut the leaves into one-inch pieces, and place in a jar of distilled water. Shake daily and keep refrigerated. It lasts two to three days. This heals so quickly it should not be used over inflamed areas that need to drain.

TEETHING

Reflexology. Work the eye, ear, and lung reflexes. Press the sides, front and back of all the toes. Rub the feet with clove oil.

Diet. Soothe the gums by giving ice cubes in a washcloth held against the gums, or cold carrot and celery sticks.

MUCUS

Reflexology. Stimulate the digestive organs, glands, and stomach. Do lymphatic and venous pump twenty five times each. Finish with effleurage fifteen times.

Diet. If babies have a lot of mucus, something is irritating them internally. Mucus is produced to help avoid or protect against an irritant. Until the mucus problem lessens, observe these guidelines:

- Avoid all grains, complex starches, and dairy products.
- Be extra careful not to overfeed, or to use salt or sugar, or to rush the child while eating.
- Make a tea, 1 tsp. each per cup of fenugreek, flaxseed, and slippery elm. Dilute with water and have the child sip, or take in a bottle, all day long. He cannot drink too much of it, and it is not dangerous in any way.
- After the problem disappears, continue to avoid all pasteurized dairy products. They are hard to assimilate, and the essential elements are rendered much less useful to the body by the pasteurization process.

Students

Students often lead a life that is not conducive to supporting a living creature. They sit, worry, eat, and do a lot of their thinking while slouching and without much enjoyment. Here are some helpful hints for this challenging situation.

STUDYING

Take a break about every hour from your reading. Remove your glasses if you wear them. Look at an object in the far distance to relax your eyes. Do some neck rotations. Stand up and stretch backward to open up the pelvis which jams with so much sitting.

Reflexology.

- Work on the big toe, and the spine and sciatic reflexes.
- Rotate the ankles, extend and flex them.
- Do thirty seconds of tapotement, followed by three effleurages.

Diet. Eat moderately while you study; digestive organs, eyes, and brain compete for the available blood and energy. Ideally it is best to study first and then eat dinner; or eat, rest, exercise, and then study.

Exercise. Bring a jump rope to school. Five minutes of this simple exercise in between classes can keep you in shape and alert. It is important that you exercise periodically when sitting so much.

EXAM TIME

Reflexology. Work all the points on your big toe, plus rotation, pull and release; do inching. Do this within fifteen minutes of an exam, or before studying for one.

Diet. Eat lightly during exams and mostly fruits and vegetables. You will be able to think more clearly and retain knowledge better. If you eat protein, stay away from fatty meats or protein with starch. Do not eat at least one hour before the exam, and do not eat white or brown sugar, white flour, or junk food during exam periods. After the initial false energy "lift" you get from them, they produce an even lower "down" than before and actually rob you of energy. Refined foods make concentration and sitting more difficult.

Exercise. After studying, and before going to bed, to aid your memory:

- Do the shoulder stand (or headstand) for one to three minutes. See photo and explanation given below.
- Do rocking ten to twenty-five times.

- Do either the reflexology wake-up exercise, in the Morning Wake-Up section, or nail-inching to the tips of all the toes and spinal reflexes.
- Then sit quietly, make sure you're relaxed, and mentally review your material without actually looking at it. End with an affirmation: "I am going to retain such and such material, and understand it thoroughly. I need not worry, it will become an integral part of my thinking." (This is good to affirm whenever you take a study break.)
- Go to sleep with no worries. Sleep is an important part of memory. It has now been discovered that certain cycles of sleep make memory possible. Get enough sleep during periods of intense studies.

Shoulder Stand.

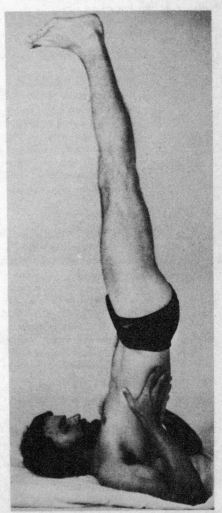

1. Lie on your back, palms facing the floor beside you.
2. Press the palms downward, as you lift your legs up and over your head. While the legs are parallel to the floor, support your back, close to your shoulders, with your hands.
3. Lift your legs, trying to come as high up on your neck as possible.
4. Make sure your body is in alignment (chin in line with navel and big toes.) Relax your feet, face, and breathing.

Shoulder stand.

Senior Citizens

It would be especially nice if the senior citizens became proficient with integrated reflexology and shared it with friends and family. They may be interested in these specific treatments to use on themselves or on friends.

POOR CIRCULATION

Reflexology.

- Work each of the joint movements on the ankles, all the toes, plus stretch the tendons.
- Do friction with the knuckles on top and bottom of feet.
- Work the entire spinal reflex, genitals reflex, all calf points, and this SPECIAL CIRCULATION POINT: It is on the outside of the thigh. You can find it by standing up straight. Let your arm fall to your side. Where your middle finger ends, touching your thigh, is the point. This promotes blood and lymph circulation, especially to the lower limbs.
- Finish with General Lymphatics, twenty-five times, effleurage fifteen times, and nerve stroke. Make an affirmation: "My circulation is improving minute by minute."

Diet.

- Upon rising, have the juice of a fresh lemon in water with a dash of cayenne pepper, or a glass of grape juice with cayenne. Use an amount small enough to be comfortably tolerated. Add a teaspoon of kelp if there is also constipation involved.
- A half hour later, for breakfast, eat either a fruit or whole grains. Millet and cornmeal are very good for both constipation and poor circulation.
- Do not eat protein after 3:00 P.M.
- Foods to focus on: seed meals, bran, yogurt, sprouts. If you can't handle roughage well, blend up some raw vegetables. If you prefer cooked ones, blend them, but still add a few raw ones to get undestroyed vitamins and enzymes. Make sure you have enough raw food each day to keep you feeling great.

Exercise.

- Walk barefoot at least an hour a day. You are never too old to go barefoot! When possible, walk on grass, sand, or even pebbles.
- Do foot exercise. Roll your feet over a broomstick on the floor. Pick up

objects with your toes. Walk on the sides of your feet, on just your toes, then just on your heels.

● Religiously do arm swinging and neck rotations morning and night.

Arm Swinging. Stand up straight. Swing one arm in as large a circle as possible and as fast as you can. Do this first by swinging forward, ten to twenty-five times; then repeat backward for the same count. Repeat with the other arm. You may hold the arm not being used on your hip or against a wall for balance.

Neck Rotation. Rotate your neck as slowly and firmly as you can in the following manner: three times in clockwise circles, three times in counterclockwise circles.

Make vertical figure eights as though you could draw them with your chin. Make horizontal figure eights. Write your name in the air with your chin.

Lean your head back as far as possible, then begin to bring it forward. As you do so, place your fingers on your forehead and resist by pressing back. Resistance strengthens. Bring your head all the way forward; then begin to stretch it back. And once again, resist with fingers on your forehead. Place your head all the way to one side, so the ear goes toward your shoulder. With the arm opposite that shoulder, hold the top of your head. As you try to lift your head back to center, resist the movement with the hand on the head. Repeat this on the other side.

GENERAL BODY TONER EXERCISES FOR SENIOR CITIZENS

Bear Hug.

● First stimulate the lung and big toe reflex points.
● Then sit down. Grasp your hands together in front of your chest, at the level of your heart. Elbows are out to the sides.
● Inhale deeply and lift the left elbow up as high as it will go. The right one will go down toward the floor.
● Exhale deeply and lift the right elbow up, the left going down.
● Continue alternating the elbows up and down. Repeat for one minute or until your arms become tired. Relax and repeat it again.

Body Toner. This is to be done lying down.

Squeeze your hands and feet as tightly as possible for a count of five. Then release them, and relax those parts of your body as completely as you can, for a count of five. Repeat this four more times, or until tired. This is very good to do before retiring and upon waking in the morning.

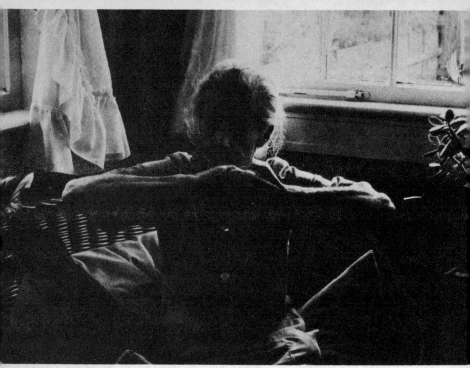

Grasp hands.

Inhale elbow upward.

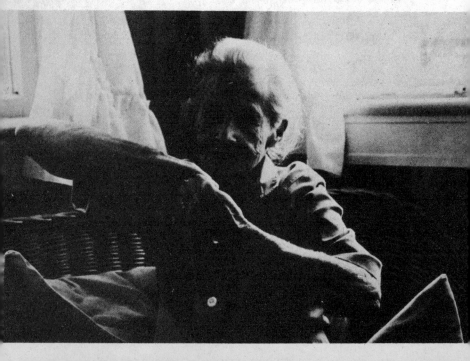

People on Their Feet a Great Deal

Our feet affect our state of mind a lot. Ever try to remain peaceful and centered, patient and loving, in the midst of aching feet and leg cramps?

Make sure you take a break for at least five minutes out of every hour. Sit down, take off your shoes (be they waitress shoes, ballet shoes, or executive specials) and socks. Let your feet "breathe" and cool off. Run your feet under alternating hot and cold water, ending with cold. (You can do this in most any restroom, if necessary.) Keep a rolling pin or some such object in your drawer. Roll your feet back and forth over it, stimulating all the reflexes, and conserving your energy at the same time. Do nail-inching and do knuckle rubbing all over the feet. Do the toe pull with release on the tendons. If you are very short on time, do just the big toe.

Then, prop your feet up on something, so they are higher than the rest of your body. Deep breathe, drawing the breath and a visualization of cooling energy to your feet. Do this three times. End with an affirmation, "I am renewed, centered, and full of life."

Return to whatever you were doing, that much the better for your five minutes of effort.

The Constructive Ten-Minute Coffee Break

This is not a suggestion to drink coffee! It is an alternative procedure, to use your coffee break time to renew yourself.

Coffee and commercial black teas contain a lot of caffeine and acids that irritate the system, wire you up with false energy that is bullied out of the endocrine glands, trap you in stimulatory addiction, stain your teeth, and wash your body of precious magnesium that keeps the colon "sweet," meaning at the appropriate pH.

ATP (adenosine triphosphate) is our bodies' form of "currency" or usable energy. It lets go of phosphate molecules to supply energy to keep cells "turned on." When rest is necessary an enzyme combines with ATP to "stop-it." Caffeine in coffee and theophylline and theobromine in black tea closely resemble adenine. They thus fool the enzyme and combine with the enzyme themselves. Thus

ATP is prevented from "resting" and we seem "turned-up and hyped-up." This constant release of energy eventually stresses and wears us down. All the way around, coffee and black teas are boogeymen to avoid.

REFLEXOLOGY

Before eating, drinking, or chatting, sit quietly for a minute to watch your breath calm down. Then take three deep breaths, using the three-part deep breathing. Do tapotement (clapping and slapping) over your entire feet and legs for one to two minutes. Finish with nine effleurages, stretching the skin firmly from your toes up to your knees.

EXERCISE

- Sitting in a chair, lean your head down toward the toes. Rap your neck, shoulders, and head firmly with your knuckles. Gently pull at the roots of your hair to loosen the scalp. All these areas naturally tense up as you sit at a desk, type, or write. This constant tension deprives your brain of nutrition and you of energy and top performance. It is very important to break up the tension.
- Lean back comfortably in your chair, and starting from your feet up, slowly rotate each joint of your body, beginning with the toes. Rotate them three times, in circles, in each direction. As you do this, mentally say to your toes, "Relax!" Then on to the ankle joints, and repeat this procedure. Continue up all your joints up to your neck. In a chair your movements may be slightly limited, but still effective. Command each joint to "Relax!"
- When you finish, make an affirmation such as: "I am full of energy. I will continue to be rested and renewed the rest of the day."

DIET

Now enjoy a cup of something to drink that will soothe and give you energy. If you insist on a stimulant, maté tea is naturally stimulating without the extensive harmful acids or additives of coffee. However, grape juice with cayenne is a completely harmless energizer. Do not fool yourself with the decaffeinated coffee "hype." The chemicals used to decaffeinate coffee are worse than the effects of whole coffee. If you want to eat, eat something light and nutritious such as yogurt, fruit, seeds and raisins, or a piece of cheese. Steer away from yogurt with a lot of sugar and artificial flavoring. Enjoy your day.

8

Special Programs (continued)

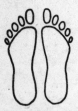

Quick Relief from Stress

We all have those times when we get angry and can't express it, or everything seems to be going wrong. Or else we become depressed for what seems like no explainable reason. You do not have to be at the mercy of stress; you can help yourself become cool and centered again. Here is a program that will help in just five minutes.

- Immediately focus on your breath. Slow it down.
- Sit down if possible and take three deep breaths, drawing them into your solar plexus.
- With each exhale, mentally say to yourself, "Relax!" Feel that each exhale is draining your tension away.
- Press both coping reflexes, between your second and third toes.

Hold them while you take three more deep breaths as above.

- Press both solar plexus points while taking three more deep breaths.
- Now place the fingers of both hands on the top of your head. Inhale deeply. On a strong, hissing exhalation, press your fingers down, and stretch the scalp downward toward your ears, as though you are trying to "dig" a little dent in the top of your head. Repeat three times.
- Inhale deeply, and on another strong, hissing exhalation stretch your face as widely as possible.
- Inhale deeply, and on another strong, hissing exhalation, squeeze your face as tightly together as possible.
- Now sit back and just explore how you feel. Observe yourself as though you were across the room watching yourself from a distance. Watch yourself as though at the end of a tunnel. See yourself as the angry person, the wronged person, the justified person, the crabby person. Be objective and see how you look to yourself.
- Now another three deep breaths. Close your eyes and draw your awareness to the forehead. Project a visualization of an image of yourself, the way you would like to look handling this stressful situation. See yourself either calm and happy, or with controlled anger, telling the person what you really think. Feel good about your actions in your visualization. Once you have a clear image of this, make an affirmation that "This is so."
- Take a deep breath and return to the situation, more centered and able to be in control of it and yourself.

If you are too upset to concentrate on doing a routine, do the following exercise.

Just Be Exercise. Either sit on your heels, or in a chair. If on your heels, place your forehead on the floor. If in a chair, place your forehead down between your knees. Breathe deeply three times, saying mentally on each exhale, "Relax!" Hold this position without moving for fifteen minutes. Even if your mind is screaming, remain still and do not fidget or move a single muscle. Then slowly rise, take three deep breaths, and make a healing affirmation.

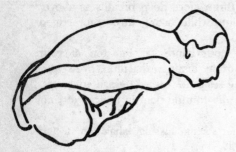

Just Be Exercise, first position.   Just Be Exercise, second position.

Do not eat or drink anything while you are upset. Get yourself and your breath centered first.

You might be asking yourself, "What is the solar plexus, and why is it so important?" Stimulation of the solar plexus reflex is an excellent aid to soothe emotional upset. This is because the solar plexus, called the *hara* ("what you are") by the Japanese and Chinese and extending from a few inches under the ribs down toward the pubic bone and including the navel, is an important "place of power" in the body. This means that many nerve centers affecting the balance of body and mind reside here. It is also the seat of spiritual centers, called *chakras*.

On the foot, the solar plexus reflex is under the lung area, in a V-like junction. When stimulating the solar plexus reflex, use both hands and hold both points on the two feet at the same time. You can also hold your hand on their solar plexus, and stimulate it by rocking your hand back and forth. Do not rub; just hold your hand and place and rock. This, and alternate stimulation of reflexes on the feet (solar plexus, coping, kidney and adrenal) calms people in mere minutes, and reduces upset, trauma, and shock. (The kidneys are the "seats of courage" and the adrenals are stressed in times of duress.) Continue stimulation until the person completely relaxes and feels pleasant.

Before giving a complete Integrated Treatment to a very high-strung person, hold the coping reflex for a minimum of one minute. The coping reflex decreases distress, depression, and even helps regain lost consciousness due to fainting or accident.

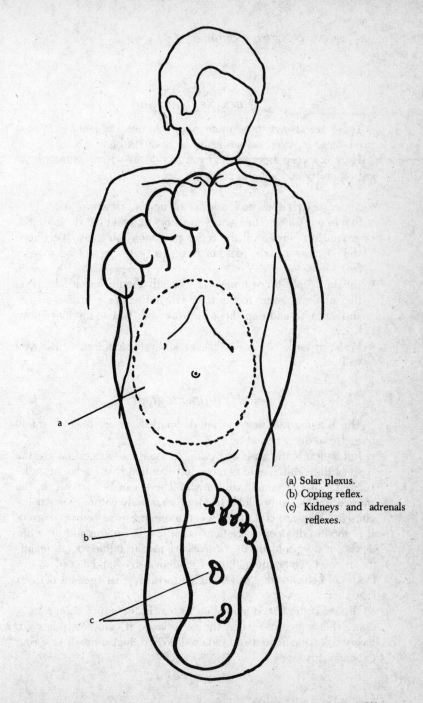

(a) Solar plexus.
(b) Coping reflex.
(c) Kidneys and adrenals reflexes.

Quick Rejuvenation

There are always those moments when one suddenly feels very tired, lacks energy, and wishes to be home in bed.

Here is a very short method you can do anywhere without looking too nutty and yet still get a lift:

- Squeeze your toes back and forth, up and down in your shoes five to ten times. Then slap your shoes and feet flat down on the ground, to percuss all the reflex points on the soles. Bang your shoe against a curb, rock, or desk, to send more blood to your feet.
- Inhale deeply three times. The breath should be visualized on the inhale as going to the feet. On the exhale visualize energy and strength and pep shoot up from your feet to fill your entire body.
- Walk onward. No one will ever know the difference. But you will!

Relaxation Program

This is a program that you can do yourself, or use to guide someone else to deep relaxation.

Relaxation is the basis of health; tension and congestion are the basis of ill health. There is more to relaxation than "seeming to be relaxed," or not emotionally upset. There can be tension on the muscle, organ, and cellular levels of your body without your being consciously aware of it. Thus, even if one presumes one is relaxed, it is good to do deep relaxations often just to tune in and tune up.

Also, many problems in our lives are manifestations of our inability to relax. Overeating, binges of depression, and boredom are modes of behavior that can be helped with regular sessions of deep relaxation.

The cat is the fastest animal on its feet in the entire animal kingdom. This is because when the cat relaxes, it completely lets go. Every cell is nourished and repaired. When the cat needs to spring to action, it's ready.

Are you ready to spring to action after resting or sleeping? You should be if your relaxation is complete.

REFLEXOLOGY

- Hold both solar plexus points for thirty seconds. Then repeat with the coping reflexes.
- Gently stimulate the adrenals, pituitary, and cervical spine reflexes.
- Do gentle tapotement for thirty seconds. Done this way, tapotement becomes sedative. Then end with three gentle nerve strokes.

DEEP RELAXATION

This directly follows the foot reflexology treatment:

- Lie down or lean back in a comfortable chair.
- Take five deep breaths. Feel yourself let go of all tension.

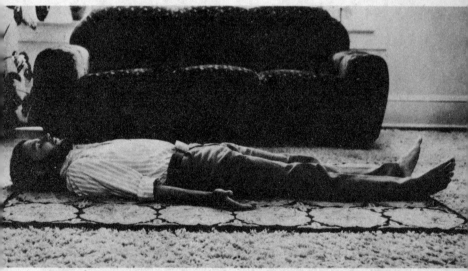

Deep relaxation. Lie in a corpse pose, flat on back with palms up toward ceiling. Can also be done in a chair.

- Draw your awareness to both feet. Inhale a breath to your toes, arches, heels, to the entire foot. On the exhale, mentally say to yourself, "Feet Relax!" Repeat this mentally three times. Try to visualize all cells, blood vessels, and muscles relaxing. Picture this in a way that seems plausible to your imagination.
- Continue this same procedure for the following areas of your body: legs, knees, thighs, buttocks, reproductive organs, lower back, middle back, upper back, shoulders, arms, elbows, forearms, hands, abdomen and abdominal organs, chest, heart, lungs, neck, face, head, brain, eyes. Draw a breath to each area and on the exhale, command and visualize that area relaxing.
- Now forget about your body and draw your awareness to your thoughts. Think of your mind as a blank screen. Your thoughts are merely colorful images that flash on and off that screen. Observe your mind as an objective witness, a person sitting in a theater objectively watching a screen.
- Begin to observe the spaces between the thoughts, the moments when the screen is blank. Become very aware of the blank spaces as though you could dive deep into them, beyond the images or thoughts.
- Rest deep within, beyond your body, mind, or breath. Stay this way for anywhere from thirty seconds to whatever time period is comfortable. At first this may seem difficult to do, but mentally discipline yourself to do it, and soon it will be easy.
- When you become active again, take a few deep breaths.
- Slowly move your fingers and toes. Stretch out, twist from side to side.
- Slowly sit up. Be thorough about being slow. Transitions are important. Throughout the day, be gentle with your transitions. From sitting to standing, from eating to working, be smooth. Make an affirmation. An example is: "I am full of energy. I am renewed." Have a nice day.

Deep relaxation is not sleeping. It is more powerful than sleep if done properly. When you are first inhaling to each area of the body, really visualize and feel the muscles becoming soft and creamy. Feel the skin and muscles hanging limply on the skeletal structure with no resistance. Feel the organs relax and soften. This does not necessarily happen in sleep; most people wake from sleep muscularly stiffer than before.

For a more effective deep relaxation, do not allow yourself to move at all after having gone throughout the body with the breath.

Deep relaxation takes about fifteen minutes, and should be done twice a day if there is a deep problem. Relaxing is not only a time of lying down or sitting quietly, but an attitude of mind that should be practiced all day, even while being active. Short periods of re-laxation spaced throughout the day give one more stamina, efficiency, and joy from the day. One can relax while sitting in a car at a red light; one can inhale to the muscles and command them to relax while walking. When eating threatens to get out of control, instead of "binge-ing" discipline yourself to relax. Most of our binges and emotional extremes are due to tension. The ability to relax and remain relaxed is the foundation of successful health efforts.

DIET

Details for those who have trouble relaxing:

- It is very important not to overeat or to eat late at night.
- Do not eat a protein meal late in the day. Undigested protein ir-ritates the colon, producing toxins in the system that cause stress and tension throughout the body. Protein eaten before 3:00 P.M. has a better chance of being digested and completely "burned."
- Avoid all refined foods, ice, or very hot foods and drinks. Avoid falsely stimulating foods and drugs.
- Eat smaller meals and watch your food combinations.
- Do a few minutes of deep breathing and relaxation before each meal.
- Before lying down to relax or sleep, take a balanced B-complex tablet with six calcium lactate tablets. Drink down with a warm glass of raw milk, or the following teas: hops, valerian root, or catnip. You may use the teas as a mixture or singly. If no tea or milk is available, try warm lemonade or grapefruit juice.

EXERCISE

Do a lot more walking or exercising in the open air, especially before going to bed. Do deep breathing as you walk and make affirmations. Set aside five minutes, twice a day, for deep breathing. As you do it, stimulate your solar plexus and coping reflexes.

Relaxing Exercises. The following exercises should help whether performed alone or in combination:

- Lie on a slant board for fifteen to twenty minutes.
- Do a shoulder stand for three minutes. If this is difficult, do a partial shoulder stand by bringing your legs only high enough into the air to support your knees with your hands and to balance yourself.

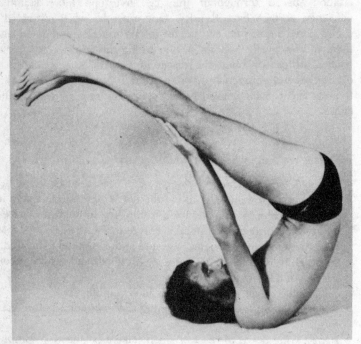

Partial shoulder stand.

- Do the Just Be Exercise in the Quick Relief from Stress section.
- Cat and cow, done twenty times before going to sleep, flexes, clears, and strengthens the spine, making it easier to relax: 1. Be on hands and knees. Inhale and arch the right leg and head up. 2. Exhale and contract your head and knee together. Repeat ten times on each leg.

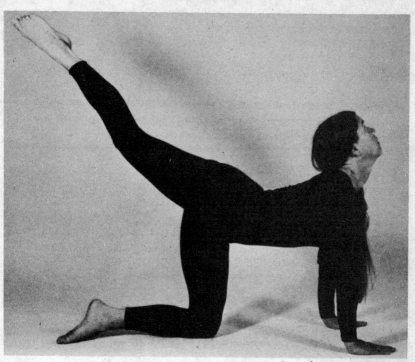

Cat and cow exercise, Step 1.

Cat and cow exercise, Step 2.

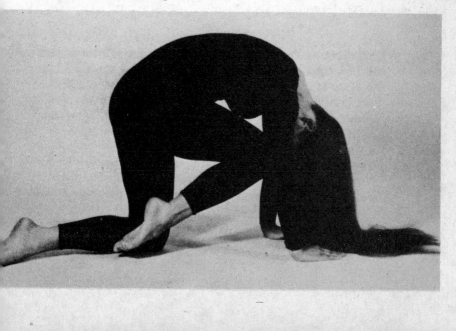

One-Month Cleansing Program

Where you start on this diet depends on the diet you are eating now. If you eat a normal American diet, start at First Week. If you are already on a light vegetarian diet, start at Second Week, and repeat for two weeks.

FIRST WEEK

Reflexology.

- Focus on all the organs of elimination: lungs, kidneys, liver, skin (the "third kidney"), and tear ducts (the last two being affected by working on the kidney and eye reflexes).
- Do toe pull with release, and nail-inching on all the toes and colon point.
- Next one minute of the lymphatic reflexes, finished by one minute of the General Lymphatics movement.
- End with venous drainage fifteen times, effleurage six times, and nerve stroke and affirmation.

Upon Arising and Retiring.

- Do inhale-exchange-release visualization to all your organs of elimination. If time permits, do it to the whole body in a deep relaxation.
- Do skin brushing, and take a shower.

Diet.

BREAKFAST: Fruit with melon at least three mornings. One half hour later you may have either one egg, a small piece of fish, 2 oz. of seeds, a small bowl of yogurt, or a piece of whole-grain toast. Starting the fifth morning, eat only the fruit.

LUNCH: 1 protein (cottage cheese, nuts, piece of fish or sesame butter; no hard cheese). Four to six steamed vegetables of varying colors, and a salad with raisins or chopped figs.

DINNER: Baked potato, yam, parsnips, carrots, or winter squash. Bowl of steamed zucchini (alternate with bowl of steamed string beans, asparagus, or beets). Large salad or Green Drink (see page 142).

LATE SNACK: Fruit or tea.

Exercise. These exercises are to be continued throughout the whole month. Do not miss a day.

- Do three-part breathing after each reflexology treatment, for three to five minutes. This is ideally done while taking a fresh-air walk.
- Do ten minutes of exercise morning and evening. Include: cat and cow at least ten times (see Deep Relaxation), stomach flapping, Reflexology Wake-Up or Life-Conquers-All Exercise, and rocking on the spine (see Morning Wake-Up).

SECOND WEEK

Reflexology. Do the same as First Week but add:

- Stimulate adrenals, thyroid, and pituitary, in this order, before all other reflexes.
- Do one minute of tapotement before the General Lymphatics movement.

Diet.

BREAKFAST: Fruit, with melons every other morning. Do not include bananas or dried fruit.

LUNCH: Large bowl of lettuce (not Iceberg) with sprouts and at least two other vegetables, 1 cup of yogurt, or 3 oz. of seeds, or 3 T. of sesame butter. One bowl of steamed zucchini, alternated with collard greens, kale, mustard greens, broccoli, or brussel sprouts.

DINNER: Fruit salad. Optional: raisins, honey, bran flakes, shredded coconut, dried fruit bits.

LATE SNACK: Fruit or tea.

THIRD WEEK

Reflexology. Same as second week except add venous drainage, twenty-five times.

Diet.

First, Second, Third Days.

BREAKFAST: Liver Flush Drink (see page 163) followed by glass of warm water or tea.

LUNCH: Fruit, no more than three kinds per meal, melons alone.

DINNER: Large raw salad with sprouts and dried fruit bits.

Fourth, Fifth, Sixth Days.
BREAKFAST: Juice (only fresh).
LUNCH: Fruit (preferably melons, or apples, or citrus in season, or grapes).
DINNER: Melons alone, or apples
LATE SNACK: Lemon and honey in water or tea.

Seventh Day. All day water fast. (If this is too hard for you, add lemon and a little honey to the water.)

FOURTH WEEK

Reflexology same as third week.

Diet.

First Day.
BREAKFAST: Diluted juice (mixed with equal amount of water).
LUNCH: Melon or apples.
DINNER: Melon or apples.

Second Day.
BREAKFAST: Liver Flush Drink.
LUNCH: Three pieces of fruit.
DINNER: Small bowl of lettuce and tomatoes.

Third Day.
BREAKFAST: Fruit.
LUNCH: Salad with sprouts.
DINNER: Salad and steamed vegetables.

Fourth Day.
BREAKFAST: Fruit.
LUNCH: Large salad with sprouts. Dressing or side dish containing yogurt or sesame butter.
DINNER: Baked potato or yam, steamed vegetable, and homemade soup (not creamed) or salad.

Fifth Day.

BREAKFAST: Fruit. Optional: one half hour later, 1 oz. seeds or bowl of sprouts and raisins.

LUNCH: 1 cup yogurt, or cottage cheese, or 1 egg or 1–2 oz. seeds. Bowl of steamed vegetables or large salad.

DINNER: Soup and salad, steamed vegetables and millet, or sauerkraut. Salad may have raisins or chopped figs in it.

Sixth Day.

BREAKFAST: Fruit. Optional: one half hour later, 1 oz. seeds, or egg, or bowl of sprouts.

LUNCH: 3 oz. seeds, or egg if not eaten at breakfast, or 4 oz. fish, with vegetables, cooked or raw.

DINNER: Steamed vegetables plus baked potato or yam or buckwheat groats or brown rice. Optional: pickles made without sugar, salt, or additives.

Seventh Day.

BREAKFAST: Fruit, or millet or whole oatmeal, or blend some soaked raw grain with apples, raisins, honey, and cinnamon.

LUNCH: One protein (anything but red meat and turkey), plus four to six steamed vegetables and salad.

DINNER: Homemade soup, slightly sautéed vegetables with yogurt dressing (mix yogurt and sesame butter, for which 2 T. of tofu can be substituted, with 1 T. oil, 1 T. vinegar, spices—dill, garlic, kelp.)

Slowly begin to introduce new food. For another week carefully watch your menu before you resume a heavier diet. Throughout the four weeks, drink this *Citrus Water* throughout the day, as well as upon arising and retiring: 1 gallon of water with 10 lemons freshly squeezed, 2 oranges, and 2 grapefruits. If desired, add a little honey. When making the salad dressing, you may blend in a few whole vegetables such as celery, tomato, avocado, carrot, to make it thicker and tastier.

Fourteen-Day Reducing Program

FIRST WEEK

Reflexology.

- Intense stimulation of thoracic spine reflex (sympathetic nerve stimulation causes a mobilization of fat!)
- Stimulate all glands, including pancreas, and genital reflexes.
- Nail-inching on all toes and colon point.
- Tapotement one minute, followed by all lymphatic points, effleurage, and nerve stroke.

Diet.

UPON ARISING: One glass of *Gland Drink:* 1 T. granular kelp, 1 tsp. powdered rosehips, and ¼ tsp. cayenne. All three together act as gland revivers (special healing recipe from Eva and Gene Graf, Connecticut).

BREAKFAST: Fruit only.

LUNCH: All the steamed vegetables and salad and sprouts you can eat. Dressing should have at least 2 T. of cold pressed vegetable oil. Add 2 oz. seeds, or 1 egg, or 4 oz. fish (fresh water).

DINNER: Choice of fruit or vegetable meal. Fruit: Enjoy 3–4 pieces of whole fruit, or cut up with 4 T. yogurt, or 2 T. shredded coconut, or 2 T. sesame butter, ½ tsp. cinnamon plus 1 T. currants. Vegetable: Large salad with at least three types of green vegetables. Steamed vegetables excluding parsnips, carrots, yams, and winter squashes. Can make dressing or sauce with 2 T. sesame butter, 1 tsp. organic soy sauce, 2 T. yogurt, 1 clove garlic, juice of one lemon, ½ tsp. tarragon or sweet basil, and blend.

SNACKS: Fruit, tea or bowl of sprouts with no more than 15 raisins.

Do not use butter. Mix ¼ cup butter plus ¾ cup cold pressed safflower oil in blender. Saturated fats need to be combined with unsaturated fats, or they cause fat build-up in the body.

Whenever thirsty, drink distilled water, tea, or Citrus Water (page 121); do not sweeten.

Exercise.

- Morning and night, do shoulder stand for three minutes, rocking on the spine twenty-five times, cat and cow ten to twenty-five times (see Deep Relaxation), neck rotations (see Senior Citizens), woodchopping exercise (page 130), and *thyroid tapping:* Sit erect and turn your head to the right. With your right hand tap the left side of your throat and thyroid, while saying "Ah" out loud. Repeat on other side.
- Every night do deep relaxation without fail. This decreases the anxiety and escape emotions that are powerful causes of overeating. Every time you desire to binge, force yourself to do a deep relaxation, ending with a visualization and affirmation. Get a clear detailed image of how you want to look, and affirm. "I am losing weight. I am dissolving fat. My will is strong. I am becoming trim and healthy."
- Train yourself to state an affirmation first thought upon waking and last thought before falling asleep.
- Do skin brushing twice a day.

SECOND WEEK

Reflexology. Same as first week, but add calf points, venous pump fifteen times after tapotement, and General Lymphatics fifteen times.

Diet

UPON ARISING: Gland Drink.

BREAKFAST: Juice—fresh.

LUNCH: Raw salad with 3 T. raisins or chopped figs, steamed vegetables (make sure you have 2 T. oil).

DINNER: Raw vegetable or fruit salad.

NIGHTTIME TODDY: Blend the pulp and juice of 1 lemon with 1 glass of warm water and 2 T. honey.

Slowly return to a heavier diet. Each day introduce a new food, but do not revert to bad habits.

Recommended: I would suggest an enema the first three nights of the second week to speed up weight and toxin loss. Soak in hot tub with two pounds of epsom salt, three nights a week, both weeks, for the same reason.

9

How to Use
Reflexology for
Common Ailments

. . . that shouldn't and needn't be common

Anemia
Arthritis
Asthma
Back Problems
The Common Cold
Complexion Problems
Digestion Problems (including constipation)
Double Chin
Eye Problems
Hair Problems
Headaches, Dizziness
Heart and Circulation Problems

Presented here are specific health ailments with outlined programs of shortened treatment in reflexology, diet, exercise, visualization and affirmation techniques. These programs are variations on the Integrated Treatment and are designed to help relieve a problem that already exists and to prevent a problem from occurring.

Unless otherwise specified, it is understood that the reflexology treatments are to be done for five minutes morning and night, with all strokes done at least three times. The exercises are to be done ten minutes morning and night so the body has the benefits of the special elements in the air at those times.

Caution: When beginning any new diet or exercise program, start moderately and gently, avoiding extremes. Have a transition period. Guide yourself by your own feedback, by love and respect for yourself.

Anemia

REFLEXOLOGY

Stimulate spinal reflexes, all glands, liver, and digestive organs, and spleen. Do nail-inching in lung areas, working deep under the fatty pads or calluses and hooking your fingers up and under if need be. Do General Lymphatics and nerve stroke fifteen times each; then a healing visualization and affirmation.

DIET

Emphasis is on alkaline fruits and vegetables. Avoid coffee and commercial tea, making sure you don't have them two hours before or after an iron supplement or a meal high in iron. (They combine the iron with tannic acid for a ferrous tannate that your body can't use.)

Foods to emphasize: parsley, bananas, dark leaf greens, raisins, apricots, beets, seeds, egg yolks and liver, yeast, sprouted grains. All berries are especially good. Suggested teas: dandelion root, raspberry leaves, and comfrey. Suggested supplements: balanced B-complex, up to 500 grams of Vitamin C, manganese supplement, organic iron (small amounts).

EXERCISE

- All respiratory exercises.
- All liver exercises.
- Deep breathing, long walks, spinal rocking

Arthritis

REFLEXOLOGY

Stimulate big toe, all digestive organs, spine. Stimulate areas that correspond to painful arthritic areas. Special attention: pituitary, thyroid and parathyroid glands, stomach, small intestine, colon.

Do all lymphatic strokes very firmly ten times, venous pump three times, effleurage three times, nerve stroke three times. Make positive affirmations at least three times a day.

DIET

Absolutely no animal foods at all except yogurt (go on a cleansing diet to make a transition to vegetarian diet). If you are going to switch to vegetarian diet after a heavy meat diet, take at least four to six months. Absolutely no coffee, sugar, salt, or alcohol. Substitute honey and kelp.

Emphasize green vegetables, cooked or raw. Especially good are sprouts, potatoes, parsley, garlic, comfrey, bananas, pineapples, and sour apples.

Suggested supplements: alfalfa tablets; 1 qt. alfalfa seed or comfrey leaf and root tea daily; ½ cup liquid acidophilus with each meal; bromelain (pineapple enzymes), two tablets with each meal; balanced B-complex; 2 bowls sprouts daily; 2 T. brewer's yeast three times a week; 6 garlic capsules daily.

Fasting has the best result with arthritis; fast on water or vegetable juice, or raw potato juice. There are many good books on fasting.

Raw goat's milk and its products may be tolerated a few days a week. Experiment with your own feedback. If you feel good eating it, continue. If your arthritis flares up, avoid even goat's milk.

If you presently take large amounts of drugs, withdraw slowly, and take large amounts of Vitamin C. Tea for pain: valerian root.

DAILY RECOMMENDATIONS

- Each day skin brush and take hot and cold showers, and expose your eyes to sunlight for at least twenty minutes, even on a shady or rainy day. Take off your glasses. (Studies show people with glasses, which decrease ultraviolet exposure to the eyes, have higher rates of arthritis.)
- Castor oil packs on non-inflamed joints; rub grated onion, garlic and potato into inflamed joints.
- Massage body daily with oil made of ¼ mustard, ¼ peanut, ¼ olive, and ¼ castor oil.

EXERCISE

- Do joint rotations mentioned in Constructive Ten-Minute Coffee Break.
- Develop your abdomen and lungs through exercises mentioned in Digestive and Respiratory sections. This is very important.
- Take open-air walks.
- Lie on slant board fifteen to twenty minutes, twice a day.
- Do as much spinal rocking and Reflexology Wake-Up Exercise (see Morning Wake-Up) and as many shoulder stands (see Students) as possible.
- Do breath and visualization strokes into painful joints.

Asthma

REFLEXOLOGY

Stimulate all toe points, nail-inching on all toes. Stimulate bronchials, lungs, and all lymphatic drainage points. Stimulate entire spine very thoroughly; also all glands, especially adrenals, and stimulate solar plexus. Sedative tapotement (gentle). Effleurage fifteen times. Ten to fifteen nerve strokes. Healing affirmation.

DIET

Avoid all heavy proteins and any cow's milk products. A vegetarian-oriented diet is best. Avoid all starches, flours, sugars (even dried fruit and honey). Eat a lot of sprouts, goat yogurt, onions, garlic, greens, and horseradish.

Fast one day a week on juice, preferably a mixture of carrot, beet, and apple or carrot and parsley, or go on One-Month Cleansing Program.

If attacks are frequent, add these daily supplements: 200 mg B_6, 3 T. brewer's yeast, 2 tsp. crude pollen, 1 T. apple cider vinegar and 1 T. honey in warm water, three times a day.

Teas. Comfrey, lobelia, mullein, skullcap. Comfrey is important to eat in large quantities, at least 5–6 tsp. a day. You may also use the dried herb, a few tsp., as a salad herb, or powder it and put into gelatin capsules.

Chest packs. Soak flannel in warm mixture of ½ apple cider vinegar and ½ honey. Wring out and place on chest. Repeat when pack becomes cool.

EXERCISE

A must: Deep breathing for five minutes two to three times a day. Deep relaxation two times a day. The following three exercises are to be performed morning and night.

Asthma Exercise 1. Stretch back, keeping the toes forward, thus stimulating the reflexes. Spread shoulders widely and downward, pushing chest upward toward ceiling. Breathe deeply five times. Repeat five times.

Asthma Exercise 2. 1. Inhale as you sit on heels and clasp hands behind back. Pull shoulders back to open chest to take a very deep breath. 2. Next, exhale forward, stretching arms above head and in front of the body. Exhale very completely. Rise up and repeat fifteen times.

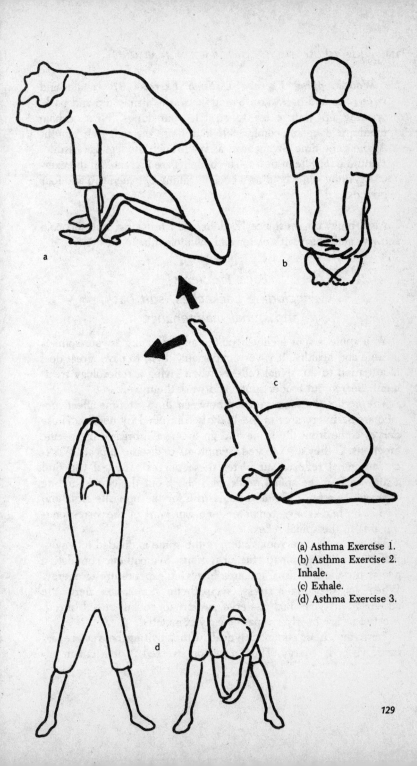

(a) Asthma Exercise 1.
(b) Asthma Exercise 2.
Inhale.
(c) Exhale.
(d) Asthma Exercise 3.

Woodchopping Exercise (Asthma Exercise 3). Inhale and stretch up and backward. Swing your arms firmly, up and back, opening up your chest to stretch your lungs. Next, exhale loudly, making any comfortable loud noise through your mouth. At the same time, swing arms as far through the legs as possible. Continue for fifteen times. The benefits are increased if the exercise is done while holding a book weighing between two and four pounds.

Also, build up resistance by doing skin brushing, hot and cold shower, and finish with castor and olive oil rub.

Back Problems
. . . including backaches, stiff back,
and spinal maintenance

Your spine is your lifeline. You are only as young as your spine is flexible and healthy. It is very important, then, to pay a great deal of attention to the spinal reflexes when giving a reflexology treatment. Search out tender spots, and work them well.

The nerves that emerge from between the vertebrae affect specific areas. Every area of the body is controlled by nerves. These nerves come from the spine and go to specific organs for specific functions. If they are blocked, symptoms of disease appear. Working on spinal reflexes stimulates these nerves. Thus, if you find a sore area on the spinal reflex, also check out the corresponding organ at its reflex. This also holds true for the opposite situation: if you later find a congested or tender organ, work on the corresponding area in the spinal reflex.

The autonomic nervous system of the spine is divided into sympathetic and parasympathetic subsystems. Sympathetic stimulation affects the thoracic area, the area involving expenditure of energy. When you are under stress, sympathetic stimulation alerts the adrenals and your body's nerve system to go full speed ahead. Most of us are overly sympathetically stimulated.

Parasympathetic stimulation deals with activities that restore and conserve body energy. Thus, a person stressed is deficient in en-

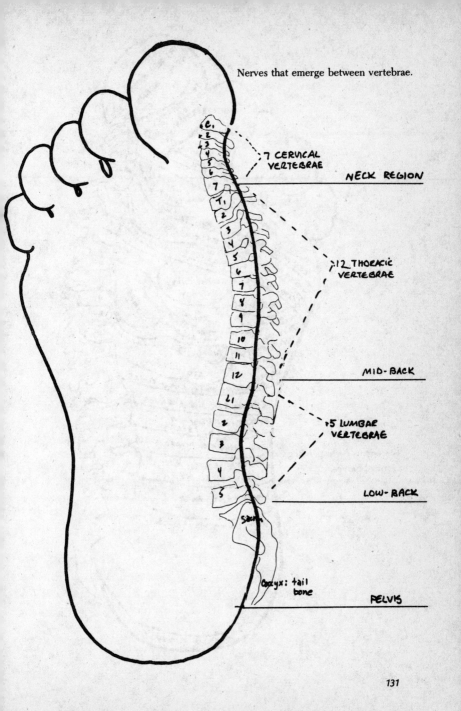

Nerves that emerge between vertebrae.

7 CERVICAL VERTEBRAE

NECK REGION

12 THORACIC VERTEBRAE

MID-BACK

5 LUMBAR VERTEBRAE

LOW-BACK

Coccyx: tail bone

PELVIS

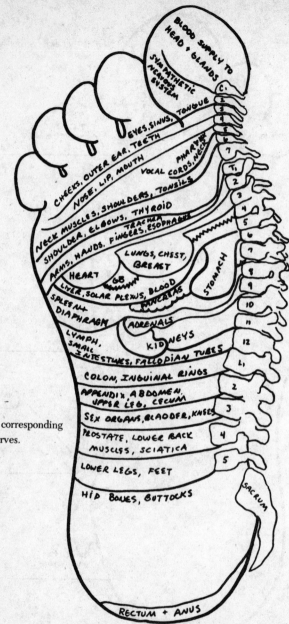

The organs corresponding
to spinal nerves.

ergy; so stimulate his parasympathetic centers by working the cervical and sacral spinal reflexes.

When people sit a great deal or get too little exercise to restrict movement in their hips, work the lumbar and sacral reflexes well. Many large and small nerves branch out from them; energy flow to the hips, genitals, and lower limbs is easily blocked by tension and stiffness.

BASIC BACK TREATMENT FOR STIFFNESS AND PREVENTIVE MAINTENANCE

Reflexology. Work all spinal reflexes in detail. Also big toe release, and all big toe contacts. Rotate big and little toes. Do plexus pull and ankle rotation (all variations). Work corresponding organs to sore spots on spinal reflexes. Do lymphatic effleurage, tapotement, venous pump ten times, effleurage three times. Then nerve stroke and healing affirmation.

Diet. When you have a backache:

- Eat less.
- Eat less protein.
- Do not eat late at night.
- Make sure your bowels are moving freely.
- Eat at least one huge green salad a day.
- Fast on vegetable juices once a week, especially beet, carrot and apple mixed together.

Herbs for Backache Pain. Yarrow, burdock root, and comfrey, to keep your system cleansed. Valerian root and willow bark for pain. A painful back could indicate a tumor or disk problem, among several other possibilities, and your physician should be consulted. If he or she does not recommend a conflicting, personalized treatment for such a specific, I would recommend taking a balanced B-complex vitamin, with six calcium lactate tablets. Chew the tablets well and take with a cup of valerian and willow bark tea, mixed with raw milk, sweetened to taste.

Exercises to Strengthen and Limber the Entire Spine.

- Spinal rocking (see Morning Wake-Up).
- Cat and cow (see Deep relaxation).
- All the exercises to open up the pelvis (Exercises 6 through 9 for Lower Backache).

- All the exercises for lower-back pain.
- Jumping rope for five minutes a day stimulates the entire spine and cere-bro-spinal fluid, and increases the cellular nutrition to all parts of your body.

LOWER BACKACHE

Reflexology. Focus on all lumbar and sacral points. Do spinal twist, ten times. Do all ankle movements, five times each. Work sciatic nerve (use a pencil eraser to get deep into it if you need to), hips, knees, genitals and kidneys. Work all lymphatic points. Venous pump ten times. Effleurage five times. Do nerve stroke and healing affirmation.

Diet.

- Eat lightly.
- Keep bowels clear.
- Eat plenty of melons or juicy fruit.
- If due to inflamed or stressed kidneys, go on a three-day watermelon diet. You may also drink, during this fast, apple and cranberry juice. When resuming eating, avoid salt and heavy meats (e.g., red meats, fatty meats).

Herbs. Mistletoe and willow bark. Burdock root and kinnikinic (*uva ursi*). Watermelon seed tea (simmer for twenty minutes).

Exercise. Do any three of the following exercises in the morning and another three at night: 1. Cat and cow (see Deep relaxation), 2. spinal rocking (see Morning Wake-Up), and any of the following exercises 3 through 10. Exercises 3 through 6 are excellent for sciatica and lower backache.

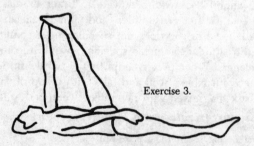

Exercise 3.

Exercise 3. Keep knees straight. Stretch toe down toward body. On the exhale, try to pull leg a little further. Hold the toe stretched down for a count of fifteen. Slowly increase length of count. Repeat three times on each leg.

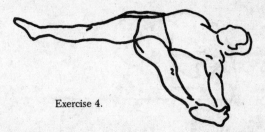

Exercise 4.

Exercise 4. Keep both knees straight. Pull toe of outstretched leg toward body. To heighten stretch, turn face in opposite direction of outstretched leg. Hold for count of fifteen. Repeat three times on each leg.

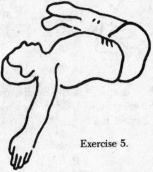

Exercise 5.

Exercise 5. Inhale while moving both legs to the left. Exhale both legs to the right. Keep knees straight and legs together. Repeat ten times on each side.

Exercise 6. Hold leg up. Keep knee straight. On the exhale, pull the toe downward. On the inhale, relax the foot. Repeat ten times on each leg.

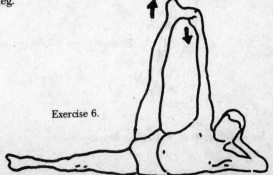

Exercise 6.

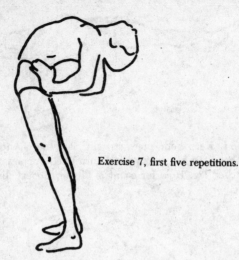

Exercise 7, first five repetitions.

Exercise 7. Inhale deeply. On the exhale, push hips forward, chest up toward the ceiling, and head is back as far as possible. Keep knees straight. Repeat ten times.

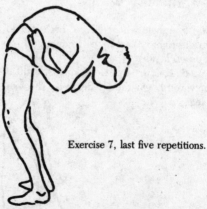

Exercise 7, last five repetitions.

Push back even further on the last five repetitions.

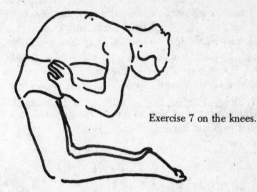

Exercise 7 on the knees.

Finally, try Exercise 7 on your knees.

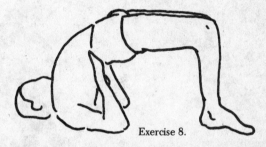

Exercise 8.

Exercise 8. First come into the shoulder stand. While supporting your back, lower one leg slowly down, and then the other until both legs are on the ground. Hold for ten deep breaths. With each exhalation, relax your lower back, hips, and buttocks even more. This is only for people who can hold the shoulder stand comfortably for three minutes.

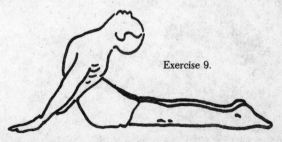

Exercise 9.

Exercise 9. Begin by lying on the abdomen. Inhale and slowly stretch chin out on the floor as far as it can go, and then lift head up and back. Push palms against the floor and raise up chest, trying to use back muscles more than the hands. Push pelvis into the floor, and then relax hips. Keep heels together if possible. Repeat three times, holding for a count of ten, with relaxed breath.

Back Exercise for Couples (Exercise 10). One person squats, while grasping hands of mate. Mate leans back, supporting weight of partner, and guides the squatting partner into doing circles in both directions, while feet remain flat on the ground. This is excellent for sciatic pain and lower backaches.

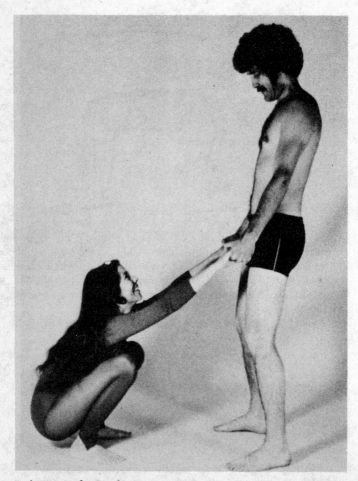

Back Exercise for Couples (Exercise 10).

The Common Cold

REFLEXOLOGY

Stimulate all toe points, toe release with tendon pull, base stretch seven times. Stimulate adrenals, spine, digestive organs, and all lymphatic points seven times. Tapotement one minute, venous pump seven times, effleurage and nerve stroke. Healing affirmation.

DIET

- Stop eating solid foods.
- Drink Citrus Water (see page 121).
- Take garlic fresh or in capsules four times a day (1 clove or 2 capsules).
- Take Vitamin C—1 gram every two hours.

HERBS

Drink freely of fenugreek, comfrey, and lobelia tea.

EXERCISE

Do shoulder stand (see Students), neck rotation (see Senior Citizens), spinal rocking, and deep relaxation. Each time you inhale to an area, visualize the oxygen opening up all the vessels and cells. On the exhale, visualize all the congestion being released. (Do this for the whole body. A congested nose is a sign of a congested body.)

At the end, visualize your whole respiratory tract, filled with white, healing, decongesting light. End with an affirmation such as, "I am clear. I am free of congestion. I am healing."

Complexion Problems

REFLEXOLOGY

Stimulate organs of digestion and elimination. Stimulate big toe, spine, and all lymphatic points. Tapotement one minute. Venous pump twenty-five times, nerve stroke. Healing affirmation.

DIET

Avoid all refined foods, especially coffee, salt, sugar, and chocolate. Avoid all cooked food and fresh food except raw goat's milk. If you insist on eating meat, stick to organ meats, fish, and eggs. Avoid all pasteurized milk products. Eat lots of raw vegetables, sprouts, fruits, seeds, nuts and whole grains.

A person with bad skin problems should go on the cleansing program, with very little or no cooked food. Every so often grate beets or raw potatoes and yams into your salads. Drink plenty of fresh vegetable juices, especially the Green Drink (see page 142).

If your diet can't be as fresh and alive as the one suggested, here are some supplement suggestions: Vitamin C—up to one gram a day; Vitamin A—50,000 to 75,000 units for two months, wait a month, then continue with 25,000; brewer's yeast—3 T. a day (Try buttermilk yeast. It's very tasty. Even as a dressing.); Kelp—2 tsp. of granules a day (or use tablets); chlorophyll liquid or tablets three times a day with meals.

HERBS

Drink this tea each morning: combine ½ tsp. each of burdock root, sarsaparilla, and sassafras. If you can obtain it, a tea of Oregon grape root is a very powerful purifier. Boil two ounces in one quart water for twenty minutes. Take ⅓ cup three times a day before meals. Try to lead a more peaceful life.

HEALING ORGANIC FACIAL

Wash face well with salt and water. Use salt as an abrasive. Mix 2 T. brewer's yeast with ¼ tsp. of cayenne pepper and enough apple cider vinegar to make a super-thick paste. Then add enough drops of water or rose water to make slightly thinner. Apply on face. Let dry completely. Wet and wash off. (May use mixture of salt, cornmeal, or almond meal to help cleanse.) Put oil from Vitamin E capsule on dry skin. Optional: put a little oil on face, before mask. Add a little powdered lecithin to mixture. This helps resolve pimples, rashes, and poor complexion. It leaves the face rosy and pink. If you have a bad acne problem, finish by rubbing face with aloe vera gel.

ORGANIC TANNER

The best tanning agent is a bar of inexpensive cocoa butter from the neighborhood drug store.

MEXICAN BEAUTY SHOWER

For your skin to be incredibly soft or quickly healed, or if you want to rid your pores of all the poisons after a cleansing or reducing regime, try this: Near the end of your shower, turn off the water and rub your skin with a mixture of ½ cup of salt with ½ cup coarse cornmeal. Rub firmly, all over your body, including your face. For a dry skin, add 2–3 T. of olive oil and add less salt. Shower well to remove all the mixture. Finish the shower with a rub of olive oil mixed with any other vegetable oil, such as almond, avocado, or sesame. To increase healing benefits, you may add some wheat germ oil and a few ounces of castor oil. Be sure to keep the mixture refrigerated. Optional additions to mixture: ¼ tsp. of cayenne makes it more stimulating. ¼ c. almond meal makes it more nourishing.

EXERCISE

- Shoulder stand (see Students)
- Cat and cow (see Deep relaxation)
- Rocking on spine (see Morning Wake-Up)
- Facial stretch (see Double Chin)
- Thyroid tapping (see Fourteen-day reducing program)
- Reflexology Wake-Up Exercise
- The Restful Complexion Exercise

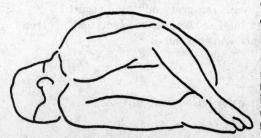

The Restful Complexion Exercise. Keep head down on the floor while sitting on the heels. Deep breathe for five minutes without fidgeting. Before rising, make fists of the hands and firmly pound lower back and back and top of head. Inhale up, stretch and then squeeze face.

Digestive Problems

The quality of your life depends on the quality of life of your digestive system. It should be clean, without pockets of hardened stools and mucus. It should be of good tone, to propel the food along. It should be clear of gas and toxins so it does not become abnormally shaped and exert pressure on other organs. All digestive problems can be helped by the following program.

REFLEXOLOGY

Stimulate the pituitary, thyroid, and parathyroid reflexes. Work the stomach, pancreas, spleen, liver, and gall bladder. Work the colon, small intestines, and anus. Give special attention to the ileocecal valve. Work all the calf points. Do tapotement for one minute; finish with fifteen effleurages, three nerve strokes, and visualization and affirmation. Watch closely for hardened deposits and tender areas. There is a good way to find these, as shown in the illustrations.

DIET

- Eat simpler, well-combined meals (see Diet, Chapter 6).
- Have a *Green Drink* at least three times a week: Mix at least three of the following in blender: spinach, comfrey, celery, sprouts, beet greens, endive or romaine lettuce. Add 1–2 cups of parsley, 1–2 T. honey, 1 T. apple cider vinegar, and fill blender up with unsweetened pineapple juice. Blend two minutes. "Chew" each mouthful.
- Foods to focus on: greens, fresh fruits, garlic, onions, potatoes, papaya, pineapple, sprouts, raw goat's milk, and yogurt.
- Each day, have large bowl of steamed zucchini, and/or green beans, and/or asparagus, and/or potatoes.

HERBS

Comfrey, fenugreek, parsley, goldenseal, cayenne.

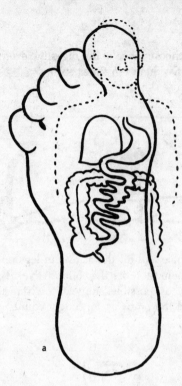

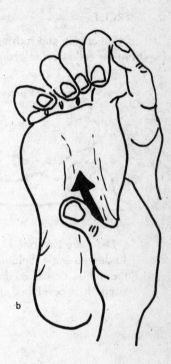

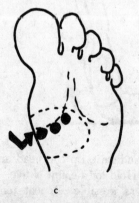

(a) A way to bring the placement of the reflexes, especially the digestive ones, to life, and make them easy to find, is to imagine the human anatomy represented on the foot.

(b) To find deposits on the digestive areas, stretch back the toes. With the thumb, firmly stretch across the instep of the foot, starting at the spine and rubbing on a diagonal. After a few deep explorations, trouble spots are easily found.

(c) An easy and effective way to get into the stomach reflex is to hook in and under the ball of the foot with your fingers. Then repeat with the thumb.

EXERCISE

Upon arising and retiring, choose three of the digestive exercises from the following selection. Do them ten times each.

Digestive Exercise 1.

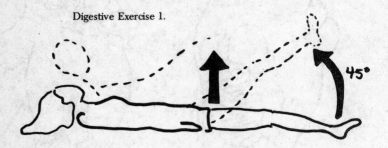

Digestive Exercise 1. Inhale and lift the arms and legs up at a 45-degree angle, holding them there for the count of five. Exhale the limbs down as slowly as possible. Repeat ten times. As strength is developed, hold the limbs up for longer counts.

Digestive Exercise 2.

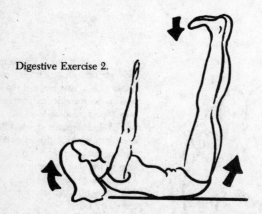

Digestive Exercise 2. Inhale and raise up the head and legs and stretch the toes downward. Hold for a count of five. Exhale while coming down as slowly as possible. Repeat ten times.

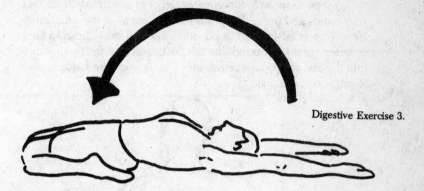

Digestive Exercise 3.

Digestive Exercise 3. Sit between heels. Lie back so the knees still rest on the floor. Inhale and raise the arms over head onto the floor. Exhale and briskly bring arms to the thighs. Keep this up at a rapid pace for twenty-five times.

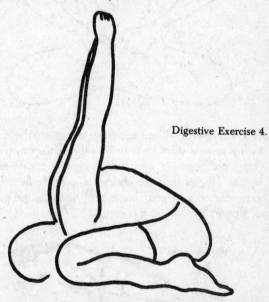

Digestive Exercise 4.

Digestive Exercise 4. Sit on heels with head to the floor. Hold arms over head and breathe deeply. Hold for three minutes.

Digestive Exercise 5. Sit cross-legged or in a chair. Makes fists of your hands and press them into the abdomen on the exhalation. Next, lean as far forward as possible, the goal being head to floor or knees. Remain relaxed like this, with constant gentle pressure into the abdomen, for one minute. This is excellent before meals to improve digestion.

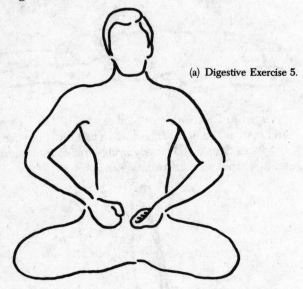

(a) Digestive Exercise 5.

Digestive Exercise 6. Place hands together on the floor with fingers facing toward your feet. Bring elbows together, and rest the abdomen on them. Lift up head, the entire body weight supported by the elbows into the abdomen and the feet. To make this exercise easier, rest your knees and head on the ground so they also support the body's weight.

(b) Digestive Exercise 6.

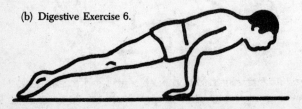

Stomach flapping twice a day is a must. Also, lie on a slant board for fifteen minutes, preferably twice a day.

After the evening's reflexology do a complete deep relaxation, then a visualization in which you "see" all the organs of your digestive tract relaxed and functioning well, and in the color and tone it seems to you that such healthy organs would look. Finally, make an affirmation of healing. An example is: "I am digesting and assimilating thoroughly. I am using all my food to its highest good, because my organs are in good tone and superb condition."

If you have trouble with abdominal pains, gas, constipation, or hemorrhoids, get a series of colonics from a qualified practitioner. If you can't do this, I would recommend taking enemas made from comfrey tea and one tablespoon of olive oil.

CONSTIPATION

For this rather frequent problem, we have this special regime.
Reflexology.

- Stimulate the following reflexes with your thumb in this order: pituitary, pineal, thyroid, stomach, pancreas, small intestines, colon (push the skin firmly up the right side, across the middle, down the left side), rectum, and anus.
- Do tapotement for thirty seconds, followed by all the lymphatic strokes three times, and venous pump, fifteen times.
- Repeat all the above procedures, this time using your knuckle, working in even deeper.
- If you have the time, repeat the same procedure again using your thumb. Thus, you will have worked all the reflexes three times. When you find tender points, use the breath and visualization strokes on the foot points and the organs themselves.
- Effleurage three times, nerve stroke three times. Healing affirmation. An example is: "I will get all the good out of my food, and then let it go. I relax inside, and let go." Then have a visual image of yourself light and unburdened and energetic. Visualize this clearly, and with a refreshing breath, let the image go.

Diet.

- Observe how you are eating. Make sure your attitude is relaxed, non-selfish, and that you chew thoroughly. To chew your food well is to cleanse your intestines.
- Constantly adjust your diet to the needs of your day. If due to circumstances you are less active, eat less. Avoid heavy starches, proteins, re-

fined food products, and enjoy many juices, whole grains, especially millet, buckwheat groats, and cornmeal.

- Emphasize fresh vegetables, fruits cooked and raw, sprouts, bran, yogurt, seeds, and nuts. Avoid hard cheese and pasteurized milk. If you eat meat, eat organ meats, fresh water fish and chicken rather than red fatty meats. Eat less meat and dairy products.
- Endeavor to cut down on the amount of animal protein you eat. Eat no protein after 3:00 or 4:00 in the afternoon.
- Upon arising, drink a tablespoon of granulated (not powdered) kelp in warm water. Other alternatives are freshly juiced pears or soaked raisins and figs blended in water with a little squeezed lemon juice.
- Try a glass of flax seed, bran, and honey in warm water before going to sleep. Swallow the seeds whole, without chewing the mixture.
- Mix homemade sauerkraut in with your salads.
- Make sure you get at least 2 T. of cold pressed vegetable oil a day. Olive or sesame are preferred.
- Supplement the diet with yeast, 3–4 T. a day, a balanced B-complex, and calcium-magnesium balanced powder.

Herbal Laxatives. Make a strong tea of senna pods with cascara sagrada. If you have a mucus problem also, add fenugreek seeds. Drink two cups of that tea before going to bed. Optional: try an enema made of the above tea. Another good enema fluid is 2 T. of olive oil and juice of 2 fresh lemons added to warm water. Do not use any laxative regularly so as not to get into the laxative habit.

Other Suggestions.

- Make sure you answer nature's call at the slightest knock, even if only to urinate.
- If you are irregular, sit on the toilet about half an hour after eating for at least fifteen minutes or until you evacuate. Try to cultivate regular habits.
- Place a stool in front of the toilet on the floor so your legs are raised and your organs and muscles are in a more relaxed and conducive position for eliminating. Hardy souls can stand upon the toilet in a squatting position.
- Lie on a slant board for at least twenty minutes before meals, to tone all the digestive organs and help the body deal with and rid itself of hemorrhoids.

Exercise. Exercise much more, morning and night. Walk in the open air, do a lot of deep breathing, and try to practice the exercises offered under the One-Month Cleansing Program regularly. Do stomach flapping morning and night without fail (see Life-Conquers-All Exercise).

Special Relaxation for Constipation. This consists of deep relaxation for all the organs of your digestive tract.

Lie or sit comfortably. Take a deep breath, and, as you let it out, mentally say to yourself the word "Relax." Repeat this three times.

Now draw your awareness and breath to various organs.

Draw your awareness to the throat. Inhale your breath to it, as though you could send the air right there. As you exhale, mentally command, "Throat, relax and let go!" Try to visualize what you think a healthy and relaxed throat would look like, and imagine your throat to look like this. Once it is relaxed, and you "see" a clear mental image, go on to do the same thing for each of the following organs: esophagus, stomach, small intestines, colon (all its parts), rectum, and anus. Go on to the next organ only when the previous one "seems relaxed" and you can visualize it in good condition. End with a healing affirmation.

Good digestion depends on good peristaltic action (the squeezing motion of the walls of the colon). Peristalsis moves the waste inside the colon on the right side of the body, from the ileo-cecal junction where the ileum (last section of the small intestines) meets the cecum (the first baglike opening of the colon). From there it goes upward to about waist level. Thus this part of the colon is logically called the "ascending colon."

Next peristalsis squeezes the waste across the middle section of the body in the thusly named "transverse colon," then downward on the left side via the "descending colon." To reach deep within the pelvis area en route to the rectum, the colon must make an "S" turn, which gives this section its name of "sigmoid colon" (the Greek name for "S").

Bad habits in exercise and life style decrease muscle tone and lessen the ability of peristalsis to push the wastes against gravity along the colon. This results in pockets of hardened stools, mucus, and gas, which decrease assimilation, exert pressure on other organs, and greatly deplete our health.

Reflexology can improve peristaltic action and thus help digestion and assimilation by: first doing nail-inching on the descending and then on the sigmoid colon. Next, doing inching with the thumb over the entire colon from ileo-cecal valve through to sigmoid and rectum. Repeat stimulation of the entire colon by pushing the skin in the appropriate direction with pressure from your thumb. Repeat again, with nail-inching.

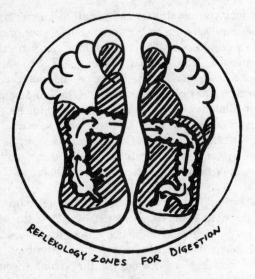

REFLEXOLOGY ZONES FOR DIGESTION

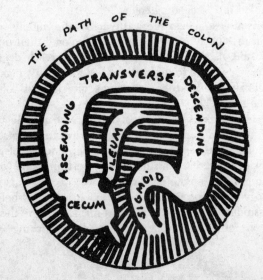

THE PATH OF THE COLON

TRANSVERSE

ASCENDING   DESCENDING

ILEUM

CECUM   SIGMOID

Double Chin

REFLEXOLOGY

Stimulate glands, spine, neck. Rotate all toes. Big toe release. Tapotement, venous pump, effleurage. Healing affirmation.

DIET

- Eat less starchy, fatty foods.
- Eat a diet of more alive foods: seeds, sprouts, vegetables, and fruits.
- Make yeast facials and put them all over chin and neck area.

EXERCISE

Neck Rotation (see Senior Citizens).

Facial Stretch. Stretch tongue down, eyes up, stretch face as far in lengthwise position as you can. Squeeze face as tightly as you can, toward nose. Alternate these two steps, five times each.

Chin Tightener Exercise. Look up toward ceiling, place fingers of both hands on forehead, above eyebrows. Try to lower head slowly while resisting with fingers pushing against forehead. (Fingers have a tendency to slip up toward hair line.) Repeat five times.

Chin Stimulator Exercise. Slap area of skin under chin with both hands. Then the area over all of your neck.

Thyroid Tapping (see Fourteen-Day Reducing Program).

Eyes

REFLEXOLOGY

Stimulate all the toes, especially the first two. Stimulate the points at the base of all the toes, especially the first two. Do toe release with tendon stretch. Do nail-inching over the entire first and second toes. Follow with toe effleurage, spine reflex, lymphatics, effleurage, and nerve stroke. Healing affirmation.

DIET

Eat a diet high in red vegetables and fruits, radishes, carrot juice, berries, kale, and yellow squash.

HERBS

Chaparral.

EYE WASHES

Slippery elm, goldenseal, and eyebright. Strain well before using. Soothing milk baths: soak cotton balls in raw, fresh milk, and cover eyes.

EXERCISE

- Sit with spine erect. Keep facial muscles relaxed and motionless.
- Inhale while moving eyes up to ceiling. Exhale down. Repeat ten times.
- Inhale eyes to right; exhale eyes to left. Repeat ten times.
- With relaxed breath, move eyes clockwise in as wide a circle as you can (see every point on the circle and keep a constant round shape).
- Do ten circles. Speed up the last five. Repeat counterclockwise.
- Focus on a close object. Then on one far away. Repeat, alternating.
- Squeeze eyes for twenty-five times as fast as you can. When you're done, let out a deep exhale. Squeeze your eyes as tightly as you can for a count of ten. Then release, rub the palms of your hands together until they are warm. Cover your eyes with the fleshy part of your palms. Let your fingers rest in your hair line. (This is called "palming the eyes.") Stroke lids out toward ears. Gently blink eyes and open.
- Make a healing affirmation for your eyes.

COMPLETE EYE REST

Palm your eyes. Keep them palmed until all you see is total blackness with no hint of light or movement. Of course your eyes are closed, but unless they are completely relaxed, it seems that your inner eye sees shadows and light. Wait for complete blackness. If it takes a while, use the exhale to help you relax the eyes more. Then blink your eyes twenty-five times, inhale, relax, and open them.

Be kind to your eyes. Whenever doing a lot of close work, take an eye break for several moments. Focus on a point far away from you; eyes relax at long distance focusing.

Hair Problems

REFLEXOLOGY

Stimulate all toes, especially big toe and big toe release. Rotate and nail-inch all toes. Stimulate all glands and genital reflexes. Lymphatic effleurage. Tapotement, venous pump, and effleurage. Healing visualization and affirmation.

DIET

Make sure you eat plenty of high silicon foods: broccoli, sprouts (especially alfalfa), comfrey, young (springtime only) horsetail plants, nettles, outer skin of cucumbers, cabbage, onions, and garlic.

Avoid salt, sugar, alcohol. Especially avoid coffee. Tests show rats on high coffee and commercial tea diets lose their hair easily. Eat seeds, yeast, nuts, leafy greens.

EXERCISE

- Shoulder stand and head stands, or handstands, or slant board two to three times a day.
- Spinal rocking.
- Massage scalp, gently pulling hair at roots.

Keep scalp very clean, don't let dandruff or dirt build up. Do not wear hats too often. If you work at a desk, or have a lot of head work and mental stress, take breaks and massage scalp. Or stand on your head in a quiet corner.

Hang your head and shoulders over edge of bed. Brush hair from back of scalp down over rest of hair. Relax in this position for five minutes.

OPTIONAL SUPPLEMENTS

Balanced B-complex, Vitamin E, homeopathic silica, and 30 mg of chelated zinc.

TEAS

Springtime-harvested horsetail (helps assimilate calcium and silicon), alfalfa, nettles.

NIGHTLY MASSAGE TO THICKEN HAIR

Virgin olive oil plus cayenne pepper. Rub into scalp well. Put towel around head, wash thoroughly in morning. Use rosemary oil and apple cider vinegar and/or burdock burrs tea as hair rinse. Follow with cool water rinse.

DANDRUFF RELIEVER

Regular rinses with vinegar and nettle tea.

DIET FOR DANDRUFF

Eat less heavy protein, don't eat late at night, and pay more attention to your food combinations.

Headaches, Dizziness

REFLEXOLOGY

Lie down, deep breathe five times while holding solar plexus. Stimulate, very carefully and deeply, all toe reflexes. Emphasize big toe and its rotation. Stimulate stomach, digestive tract, and spine. Sedative tapotement. Very strong venous pump, effleurage, nerve stroke. Do deep relaxation and healing affirmation.

DIET

No salt. Don't eat when in pain. Don't eat protein after noontime. Eat only one protein at a time. If a headache is just leaving or coming on, don't eat. If you feel a "desperate" emotional need to, eat light juicy fruits.

HERBS

Before bed, drink a cup of mandrake and burdock tea. Willow bark, mistletoe, and valerian root help relieve pain.

EXERCISE

Lean head backward against pillow or chair. Put legs up, deep breathe into solar plexus. Take an enema; when done, lie with feet slightly raised. Deep relaxation.

Headaches are usually a signal to relax and let go, and get your diet simpler and cleaner.

Heart and Circulation Problems

REFLEXOLOGY

Stimulate big toe, big toe release, toe pull with tendon stimulation (pull last two toes for thirty seconds minimum). Stimulate heart, heart valves. Do nail-inching over all toes, heart area, liver, and do lymphatic effleurage. Tapotement one minute, venous pump fifteen times, effleurage three times, nerve stroke. Healing visualizations and affirmations.

DIET

- Absolutely no salt, sugar, coffee, meat, alcohol, or smoking.
- Cut down on all high protein foods. Emphasize low sodium, low protein, low calorie, high vegetarian diet. No hard cheeses or pasteurized milk.
- In case of arteriosclerosis: absolutely no milk products. Daily suggested items: brewer's yeast, lecithin, flax seed oil, bananas, potatoes, okra and/or asparagus and apples, 0.5–1 gram Vitamin C and 100–200 I.U. Vitamin E daily. No animal fats (no butter, margarine, or hydrogenated fats). Use a few tablespoons of cold pressed vegetable oil over food.
- Do not become overweight. Diet to stay trim if necessary.
- Avoid chlorinated, fluoridated water.
- In case of heart abnormalities, Vitamin E and cytotrophic extract of beef heart tissue should be a program you work out with a licensed practitioner.

HERBS

Hawthorn berries, raspberry leaf, rue, motherwort.

EXERCISE

The following exercises strengthen the heart, but should only be done with your doctor's approval.

- Exercise That Rests Heart.

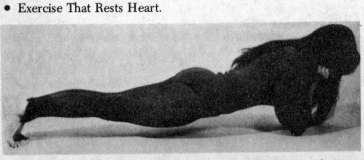

Exercise that Rests the Heart.

Lie on abdomen, place elbows on floor. Lift head, support chin with fists. Raise up so you are only on toes and elbows. Deep breathe ten times. Repeat three times.
- Slant board.
- Shoulder stand (see Students).
- Spinal rocking (see Morning Wake-Up).
- Deep breathing and fresh-air walks twice a day.
- Deep relaxation.
- Jump rope is excellent. It gets your heart rate up fast and makes you sweat. You can do it in a bathroom, hallway, outdoors, anywhere, and in five minutes you've exercised your heart really well.

10

How to Use Reflexology for Common Ailments (continued)

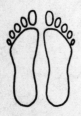

High Blood Pressure

REFLEXOLOGY

Stimulate cervical and sacral spinal reflexes (parasympathetic stimulation). Stimulate all glandular points, especially adrenals. Stimulate all kidney points, heart points, and heart valves. Sedative, gentle tapotement. Lymphatic drainage on outside sole of foot. Nerve stroke, and healing visualization and affirmation.

DIET

- Cut out sodium foods (salts, kelp, celery, romaine lettuce, watermelon, asparagus, red meats, particularly pork) and licorice.
- Eat more high potassium foods (leafy greens, oranges, potato peeling broth, bananas, seeds, and whole grains).
- Lose weight if overweight (go on reducing or cleansing program).
- Foods to focus on: garlic, onions, sprouts, seeds. Try a watermelon mono diet (eating only watermelon slices or drinking watermelon juice) for three to seven days. Eat the seeds, too, as they contain a hypotensive compound.

HERBS

Hawthorn berries, valerian root. Drink Citrus Water freely throughout the day (see page 121).

EXERCISE

- Skin brush twice a day, and take alternating hot and cold showers.
- Slant board.
- Shoulder stand (see Students), spinal rocking (see Morning Wake-Up), cat and cow (see Deep relaxation).
- Long walks, jogging.
- Deep breathing five minutes, twice a day.
- Neck rotations (see Senior Citizens).
- Do deep relaxation religiously twice a day. Just sitting and relaxing isn't enough. It must be the complete relaxation.

There are many scientific research findings that have now proven that guided relaxation programs (like the one presented here, or yoga and biofeedback) can lower mean blood pressure 20 points, mm/Hg, in a few weeks. The lowered blood pressure and healing effects which occur during deep relaxation have been found to influence the entire daily life. Studies reveal that people who practice relaxation techniques respond better to stress, keeping their blood pressure at lower, healthier levels.

HIGH BLOOD PRESSURE BREATHING EXERCISE

Do deep breathing into neck and feel the breath go to the discs between the vertebrae. Feel the breath expand the discs and lengthen the neck. Exhale out the tension. Do the same to your sacral area.

Hypoglycemia

REFLEXOLOGY

Stimulate all spinal reflexes, glands, and digestive organs. Do big toe release. Nail-inching on pancreas, adrenals, and solar plexus, fifteen times each. Plexus pull three times a day. Sedative tapotement, effleurage, nerve stroke fifteen times. Healing visualization and affirmation.

DIET

- Avoid all sweets, sugars, heavy starches, refined foods, salt, coffee, alcohol, smoking, kelp. (Too much sodium causes a drop in blood sugar.)
- Eat small, frequent meals. No more than two pieces of fruit a day.
- Take 1 T. apple cider vinegar, ½ tsp. honey in 1 glass of warm water three times a day.
- Avoid a lot of heavy protein.
- Eat two bowls of sprouts a day.
- Eat plenty of berries.
- Avoid grains unless millet or sprouted.

A Sample Diet.

ARISING: Glass of vinegar, honey, and water.

BREAKFAST: Yogurt and fruit, or soaked seeds and nuts and fruit, or millet, or an egg.

MIDMORNING: Seeds or bowl of sprouts.

LUNCH: Green Drink, steamed vegetables, yogurt (if not eaten for breakfast), potatoes or millet (if not eaten for breakfast), or fish.

AFTERNOON SNACK: Juice or tea with 2 T. yeast or bowl of sprouts and apple or grapefruit slices; or thin slice of cracker with lettuce and tomato.

DINNER: Steamed vegetables and/or salad, with: cottage cheese or millet and beans (if you didn't have any today); yogurt (if you didn't have any today); sesame butter mixed with sprouts, raisins or figs, or shredded carrots.

(All fruit juices should be diluted.)

HERBS

Drink raspberry tea daily.

SUGGESTED DAILY SUPPLEMENTS

2–4 grams Vitamin C a day, 3 balanced B-complex (1 with each meal), 2 T. brewer's yeast, kelp, B_6, B_{12}, niacinamide three times a day. If administered by a doctor, injections of adrenocortical extracts.)

EXERCISE

- Lots of fresh-air walks.
- Deep relaxation at least twice a day.
- Healing affirmations upon arising and retiring.
- Spinal rocking (see Morning Wake-Up) and shoulder stand (see Students).
- Jump rope at least five minutes twice a day.

Kidneys

REFLEXOLOGY

Stimulate all kidney reflexes, spinal reflexes, all glands. Do all ankle movements five times, and plexus pull. Tapotement, venous pump fifteen times, effleurage, and nerve stroke. Healing visualization and affirmation (especially important if kidney stones are involved).

DIET

- Low protein diet. Generous with vegetables and fruits, especially melons, papayas, bananas, and potatoes (with skins). Try three to seven days on just watermelon. Eat the seeds.
- Foods to focus on: potatoes, asparagus, parsley, lettuce, celery, raw goat's milk and products, sprouts.
- Food to avoid: beet greens, spinach (cooked), rhubarb, chocolate, coffee, sugar, tea, and alcohol.
- After meals, take ½ tsp. cream of tartar in ½ cup water. Take for four days.
- Drink this juice freely: ½ cranberry, ½ apple juice (no sugar but may add honey).

HERBAL TEAS

Kinnikinic, corn silk, watermelon seed tea (slow boil and then simmer for 20 minutes), parsley (simmer one half hour), juniper berries.

EXERCISE

- All liver exercises.
- Slant board and/or shoulder stand.
- Spinal rocking (see Morning Wake-Up).

Liver and Gall Bladder Problems

The liver and kidneys together get 49 per cent, almost half, of all available blood flow in the body; the liver alone gets about 27 per cent. It requires so much because its job is so important and it's always so busy. It maintains a temperature of about 104 degrees, due to all the activities it performs, such as detoxifying, storing sugar, etc.

The liver and kidneys are two active, principal poles of the human body, constantly purifying the system and keeping the electric life flow coursing. They must be kept healthy.

REFLEXOLOGY

Stimulate liver, gall bladder, spinal, and glandular reflexes five times each. Do all lymphatic reflexes and General Lymphatics strokes twenty-five times. Follow by stimulation of colon and Stomach 36. One solid minute of very firm, stacatto tapotement, and repeat liver, gall bladder, and spinal reflexes. Venous pump fifteen times, nerve stroke. Healing visualization and affirmation.

It is suggested that you go on a three-week liver cleansing program. The first week, stimulate twice a day. The second week three times a day, and the third week four times a day. But do not stimulate the reflexes longer than suggested; this releases too many toxins at once.

DIET

Avoid all meats except fish and chicken. Absolutely no sugar, alcohol, commercial coffee or tea, fried foods, processed foods or flours, salt, strong spices, preservatives, additives or synthetic vitamins allowed. The only canned food which you may eat freely is asparagus.

BREAKFAST: All three weeks drink Dr. Randolph Stone's *Liver Flush Drink:* Blend either 2 oranges or 2 small apples with 1 clove of fresh garlic, 1 T. olive oil, and juice of 2 fresh lemons. If you cannot use garlic, ½ tsp. of raw grated ginger root will do. Add no sweetener. The drink *must* be followed by two glasses of warm liquid, preferably herbal tea or distilled water. Do not eat any solid food until lunch.

LUNCH: Eat either fruit or vegetable meals, all you want. The first and third week you may have a small amount of protein with the lunch meal. But during the second week you eat no concentrated protein foods at all. You may have 2 T. of sesame butter with any vegetable meal.

DINNER: Fruit or vegetables. The first week you can have steamed or baked potatoes, yams, squashes, soups and vegetable casseroles, with steamed greens and salad. The second week you can have only lighter vegetables, steamed or raw, and as many of these as possible should be green. The third week you can have one slice of whole grain bread, or one piece of toast, along with the evening meal. Eat no protein, all three weeks, at the evening meal.

At both lunch and dinner, all three weeks, have 2 T. grated beets plus 1 T. olive oil, and ½ tsp. fresh lemon juice. The first night of the third week, drink a mixture made up of equal parts of fresh lemon juice and olive oil, 2 oz. each. The second night, do the same, but increase to 4 oz. each. The third morning take an enema of warm water with juice of 2 lemons and 3 T. olive oil. Follow this with lukewarm enema of freshly brewed coffee. If there is any irritation, stop treatment. If not, repeat this the fourth morning. Before bed each night, all three weeks, have two cups of strong yarrow, dandelion and parsley tea. Brew it for one half hour at least. Continue Liver Flush, every other morning, for two more months, reducing the oil to ½ tsp. the second month. Continue reflexology treatments, twice a day, for two months.

EXERCISE

To be done morning and night. However, while on the three-week program, try to do them three to four times a day.

Liver Twist Exercise. Stand with arms hanging freely. Twist vigorously from side to side. Inhale deeply as you twist to the left, exhale to the right. Twist with force. Repeat fifty times.

Windmill Stretch 1. Inhale and stretch arms up, clasping hands above head. Bend all the way to one side without leaning forward or backward, just straight to the side on a deep exhalation. Hold for five slow counts. Heighten the stretch by reaching from under the armpits. *Very slowly* inhale up. Bend to the opposite side. Repeat three times on each side.
(Illustration 10A-a)

Windmill Stretch 2. Kneel on floor, extend one leg to the side, and stretch one arm as far down that leg as possible. Next, stretch other arm over your ear to the same side as the outstretched leg. Keep elbows and outstretched knee straight. Hold this posture for ten deep breaths, feeling the organs being stretched and released of toxins on each exhalation.

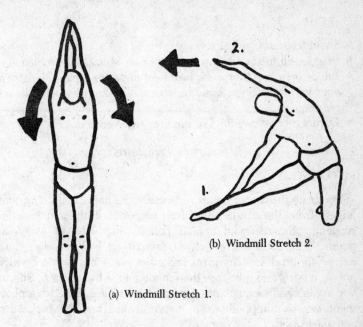

(b) Windmill Stretch 2.

(a) Windmill Stretch 1.

Low Blood Pressure

REFLEXOLOGY

Stimulate thoracics, heart, adrenals, spine, and sciatic nerve. Firm, percussing tapotement for one minute. General Lymphatic movement fifteen times. Venous pump, effleurage, and nerve stroke. Healing visualization and affirmation.

DIET

Fast only under a licensed practitioner's guidance. If he or she agrees, I would recommend eating pineapple, celery, parsley, carrots, beets, fresh grapes.

HERBS

Parsley, sassafras, and sarsaparilla tea.

EXERCISE

- Shoulder stand, spinal rocking.
- Practice all the raised hip exercises (see Menstrual Problems).
- Inhale breath to thoracic spine. Feel the discs expand, lengthen, your vertebrae align, spine become lighter and clear. Exhale out tension.
- Do deep breathing for five minutes twice each day.

Menstrual Problems

REFLEXOLOGY

Stimulate inside calf points, especially the menstrual point, four fingers from the inside ankle (see page 55). Rub, and look for swellings. Stimulate all genital points. Stimulate all glandular points. (Pay special attention to thyroid. It is like your "third ovary," for it releases thyroxine and other hormones that in essence greatly control and influence the functioning of the ovaries.) Stimulate lumbar and sacral points. Lymphatic drainage, sedative tapotement, venous pump, effleurage, nerve stroke. Healing visualization and affirmation.

DIET

- If you usually have menstrual problems, eat lightly or fast a few days before menstruation is due.
- During menstruation, make sure bowels move regularly, or take enemas.
- Eat lightly during menstruation.
- If cramps, take four to five calcium tablets, eat seed meals or sesame butter. (Also press the menstrual point, and drink valerian root tea.)
- If delayed period, drink tea of nettle, rue, and tansy.
- Be sure your diet is high in Vitamin E (seeds), unsaturated oils, calcium, B_6 (brewer's yeast, bananas, avocados, pecans, many raw foods; cooking foods destroys B_6) and kelp. If there's any doubt whether your diet provides this, take organic supplements.
- Eat yogurt, iron-rich foods, Vitamin C.
- Eat smaller, more frequent meals to keep discomfort down.

HERBS

- Excessive menstruation—ladies' mantle.
- Suppressed menstruation—life root, tansy, rue, nettle.
- Painful menstruation—valerian root, ginger root, nettle.
- Swelling—raspberry, thistle, kinnikinic (*uva ursi*).

BATH FOR CRAMPS.

Take cool water sitz baths with camomile tea plus one cup apple cider vinegar added to water.

GENERAL INFORMATION

- B_6 helps relieve swelling (100 to 300 mg a day, especially a week before period), painful lumpy breasts, and excessive flow.
- B_{12} helps restore length of cycle.
- Smoking aggravates menstrual disorder.

EXERCISE

- Spinal rocking.
- Shoulder stand. (There is controversy about inverted poses during menstruation. My experience has proven that they help relax the genital organs and soothe the body.)
- All exercises that open up hip area (see Basic Back Treatment).
- All exercises that stretch head toward knees (see page 174).
- When in pain, sit on heels or in chair. Make fists of your hands, push into ovaries on full exhalation. Lean over hands, head toward floor. Relax like this for five minutes minimum.
- Menstrual exercises.
    Step 1. Relax, while breathing deeply, for one to three minutes with legs and feet elevated and hips resting on your hands.
    Step 2. Lift up body and support lower back with hands. Breathe deeply for one to three minutes.
    Step 3. Press up with buttocks and lower back. Keep knees as close together as possible. Hold for three minutes while breathing deeply, exaggerating the exhalations.

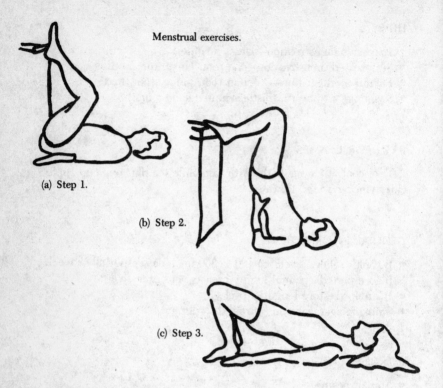

Menstrual exercises.

(a) Step 1.

(b) Step 2.

(c) Step 3.

YEAST INFECTIONS

Reflexology. Stimulate genital reflexes. Stimulate lymphatics twenty-five times. Very vigorous tapotement one minute, venous pump twenty-five times, and effleurage.

Diet. Eat garlic, yogurt, and fresh fruits and vegetables. Avoid concentrated sweets, starches, coffee, and pop. Drink Citrus Water (see page 121) throughout the day.

Herbs. Burdock, sarsaparilla and sassafras, ½ tsp. each per 2 cups water. Simmer twenty minutes.

Douche. Use ¼ cup organic apple cider vinegar to 1 quart warm water, twice a day for the first week, once a day for the second week, three times a week for the third week.

When the infection is gone, douche with yogurt diluted with water, or liquid acidophilus, three days in a row.

Pregnancy

REFLEXOLOGY

Stimulate all toes well, especially big toe and big toe release. Stimulate all spinal reflexes. Stimulate chest, breast, digestive organs. Special attention to lumbars, sacral, parathyroid, and sciatic. Do not do any nail-inching or use extreme pressure. Do lymphatics, tapotement, effleurage, nerve stroke. Do positive visualizations and affirmations at least three times a day.

DIET

- Eat fresh raw vegetables, fruits, seeds, nuts, whole grains, sprouts, tofu, goat yogurt, yeast.
- Don't overeat. Don't worry about getting enough. Just eat whole foods, chew really well, and be happy.
- Avoid coffee, sugar, salt, alcohol, and smoking like the plague.

HERBS

Take raspberry tea at least twice a day. Oatmeal water is excellent, too: ¼ cup oatmeal to 1 quart water. Simmer, covered for one half hour; strain and add honey.

Whenever constipated, take lukewarm water enema, and drink 1 T. kelp in warm water on arising.

Take no aspirins, drugs, avoid exposure to T.V. radiations, X rays, highly polluted air (including congested downtown areas of cities).

EXERCISE

- Mothers, becoming full with child, should definitely walk two to five miles *every* day. Fresh air, light on the eyes without glasses or sunglasses are very important.
- Do deep relaxation at least once a day.
- In the morning, do the following exercises (as long as possible):

Reflexology Wake-Up Exercise, polarity squat, spinal rocking, all the pelvic exercises listed under Basic Back Treatment.

- Special Pregnancy Exercise. This opens up the symphysis pubis. If practiced daily, to the point where your head comfortably rests on the floor, there is little chance of your tearing and needing an episiotomy. First, sit up straight on floor. Open legs as widely as possible. Then, inhale and stretch arms up over head. Exhale body and head forward toward the floor, between the legs. Hands and/or arms should rest on floor, with straight elbows. Hold for five counts. Then exhale, and walk fingers a little further away from you, to heighten this stretch. Inhale up. Repeat three times.

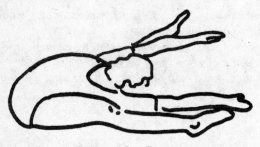

Pregnancy Leg Exercise.

- Evening exercise.
  - Pregnancy Exercise with Help. Lie on back. Draw up soles of feet so they come near buttocks, and are touching each other. Relax knees and thighs as someone presses down on the thighs. The pressure is held constant on the inhale, and deepened slightly on the exhale. Hold for one minute. Rest one minute. Hold, then rest. Build up to five minutes daily. This reduces the probability of tearing during pregnancy.
  - Pregnancy Leg Exercise. Lie on back. Lift one leg six inches off floor. While leg is lifted, rotate the ankle in circles, both directions. Then point the toes downward and hold for a count of fifteen (leg still lifted). Repeat with the other leg.
  - Shoulder stand, three minutes (see Students).
  - Cat and cow (see Deep relaxation).
  - Exercises for the lower back.

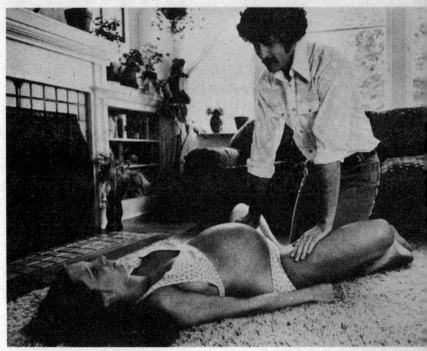

Pregnancy Exercise with Help.

GENERAL

- Your attitude should be calm, inspired, happy. The husband should encourage this. Helpful would be pictures and sayings of inspiring people throughout your home, even inside cupboards, to suprise and remind yourself as you go about daily chores.
- Please do not wear high-heeled shoes during any time of your pregnancy. It makes it difficult for your body to carry the fetus properly.
- Each morning and evening make an affirmation, with your mate if possible, about joy, health, and positive well-being for your baby. Visualize the fetus well, whole, happy. An example: "You are healthy. You are whole. You are full of light." Try inhaling energy, peace, and thanks into the new life inside you. Working with your breath, together with your baby, can be very fulfilling and calming to both of you. Have your mate do it with you, too.

Respiratory Problems
. . . including coughs and wheezing

REFLEXOLOGY

Stimulate lungs, bronchials, throat, neck, thoracic spine. Do nail-inching on all toes, lung reflex, and thoracic spine. Stimulate center of calf points. Do all ankle movements five times. Plexus pull. Tapotement, venous pump nine times, and effleurage. Healing visualization and affirmation.

DIET

Same as for asthma.

HERBS

Lobelia and comfrey.

EXERCISE

Same as for asthma. Also see Lion Pose, page 180.

Runners' and Joggers' Leg, Knee, and Foot Problems

GENERAL REFLEXOLOGY TREATMENT

Begin by stimulating Stomach 36 alternately with all the calf reflexes. Stimulate in this order feet, knee, hip, and all spinal reflexes. Rotate all toes firmly. Do flexion and extension against resistance (to strengthen peroneus longus muscle) five times. Stimulate the insertion of the Achilles tendon into the heel bone, calcaneus (see Appendix of Foot Facts). Tapotement for one minute. Venous pump fifteen times. Effleurage and nerve stroke. Healing visualization and affirmation.

LEG CRAMPS

- Work the insertions of the muscles that are cramping and the Achilles tendon insertion (massaging a muscle at its insertion into the bone it moves quickly stops the muscle spasm).
- Take 9–12 calcium lactate tablets and 200–400 I.U. Vitamin E daily.
- Eat dark leafy greens, seeds, sesame butter, and nuts; avoid pasteurized dairy products.

SWELLING IN LOWER LIMBS

- Work all the lymphatic points fifteen times.
- Follow by doing the General Lymphatics movement fifteen times, venous pump fifteen times, and effleurage three times.
- Take one gram of Vitamin C with bioflavnoids and hesperidin complex every two hours (lessen the amount if gas or acid stomach occurs).
- When swelling lessens, take 500 grams three times a day. When swelling leaves, take 500 grams a day for one month.
- Take 30–50 mg chelated zinc a day.
- Have protein at your morning breakfast, before any daily activity.

SHIN SPLINTS

- Work flexion and extension against resistance, five times each, at least three times a day. If no one can do this on your foot, try holding your foot against the wall and resisting.
- Work the lateral peroneus tendons (peroneus longus and brevis), running along the outside ankle (see Appendix of Foot Facts), by inching the thumb along them.
- Work all ankle movements.
- Very effective exercise: A week before starting a program to run, walk (with low-heeled shoes on) on outsides of feet, slightly pigeon-toed. Walk rapidly for five minutes, without stopping. When running program begins, continue this for five minutes each time before running for two more weeks. This is used by famous running coaches to help athletes with shin splints or a tendency to get them.

EXERCISE

It is important for people who regularly run and jog to keep their leg and feet muscles limbered. Also, most knee pain and injuries are due to weak foot muscles and foot and leg muscle imbalance. This can be strengthened through leg stretching exercises. Thomas M. McGuigan, practicing podiatrist and faculty member at Pennsylvania College of Podiatric Medicine, says that 80 per cent of knee problems are due to weak and tight calf muscles that pull on the knee joint.

The following exercises are for runners and joggers to help prevent injuries, for those who already have problems and want to help repair them (although you should wait until your legs are somewhat healed and not too tender), and for people who want to maintain their posture and height while aging (much height shrinkage and poor posture in older age is due to the tightening of the calf muscles).

Leg Stretch Exercise 1. Sit on the floor with legs stretched straight out in front of you, knees and feet together, backs of knees flat against the floor. Inhale your arms above your head.

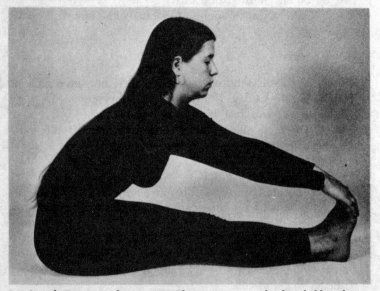

Leg Stretch Exercise 1, first position: Flexing toes, or can be done holding the pituitary reflex.

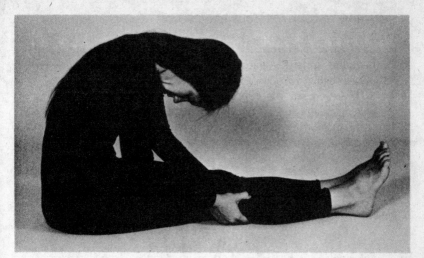

Leg Stretch Exercise 1, second position: Holding Stomach 36.

Exhale down and forward and grab the pituitary reflex on your big toes. If this is too difficult, hold either the kidney reflexes around your ankle, or Stomach 36 on the side of your leg. Relax your shoulders and head, keep your breath relaxed, and do not strain. Hold this position one minute, and slowly build up to holding it for five minutes. Before you come up, exhale fully, and stretch out over your legs as though you could touch the wall in front of you. Inhale up.

Leg Stretch Exercise 2. Stand up. Exhale down, and let your palms rest on the floor. If this is too difficult, touch each finger-tip to each toe. Hold this for five minutes, using the breath stroke to relax the calf muscles.

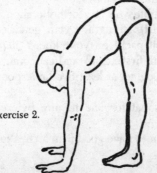

Leg Stretch Exercise 2.

Leg Stretch Exercise 3. This is for more limber people. Place the palms under the soles of the feet, hold three to five minutes, using breath stroke.

The exercises for Lower Backache are good for runners, joggers, hikers and anyone with tight hamstrings.

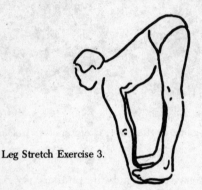

Leg Stretch Exercise 3.

SUGGESTIONS FOR RUNNERS

Do leg exercises in the morning, after the reflexology treatment, and then do a complete visualization. "See" the inner environment of your legs and feet, in detail; see the muscles limber and in good tone, and end with affirmations. Do the same thing a few hours after running, or before bed.

If you are having problems, make sure you are not running too fast, running in the same direction all the time at the track, and leaning too deeply into the curves.

If your knees trouble you, try orthotic shoe supports (you get them from a podiatrist), strengthen your quadriceps by deep knee bends, put castor oil packs on your knees (if possible, rub wintergreen oil into them first), drink and eat comfrey, kale, and parsley, and make sure you get at least two tablespoons of vegetable oil each day.

Do the polarity squat for one minute before and one minute after running.

Make sure your shoes have good firm arches to act as good shock absorbers.

Use running and walking as a time to make affirmations and deep breathe. For example, with each step say the following words: "Thank God for Life."

Sinuses, Hay Fever, Allergies

REFLEXOLOGY

Work all toes very well. Repeat the movements five times. Do all spinal reflexes and sciatic. Tapotement one minute, venous pump, effleurage. Healing visualization and affirmation.

DIET

- Stay away from all wheat, sugars, salt, flours, coffee, and alcohol.
- Drink as much Citrus Water as possible (page 121).
- Drink 1 T. vinegar, 1 T. honey in water at least three times a day.
- Suggested supplements: Vitamin C (up to 5 grams a day), balanced B-complex, Vitamin E (up to 800 I.U. a day), 1 T. crude pollen a day.
- Fast on water or juices, or do the cleansing diet.
- Eat two huge bowls of sprouts daily.
- If trouble digesting meals, try one tablet of Betain HCl after each meal.

HERBS

Black cohosh, burdock root, parsley.

EXERCISE

- Expose your eyes to sunlight at least fifteen minutes daily (taking your glasses off if you wear them).
- Shoulder stand (see Students).
- Do all the respiratory exercises.
- Do Reflexology Wake-Up Exercise morning and night.
- Sinus Exercise should be done morning and night: Lie on abdomen, arms crossed, chin rested on hands; bend knees, legs

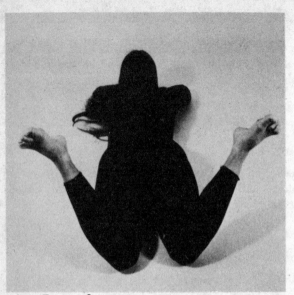

Sinus Exercise, first position.

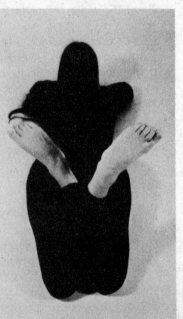

Sinus Exercise, second position.

up. Stretch legs out to side, then cross them, then out to side again. People with chronic sinus problems (congestion, headaches, etc.) should do this 50 to 100 times.

Sore Throats
. . . including bad breath, mouth sores, and sore tongue

REFLEXOLOGY

Stimulate the base of the big toe, all big toe points, rotate firmly five times in each direction, and do toe pull with release. Repeat this on all the other toes. Stimulate stomach, digestive, and spinal reflexes (including nail-inching on the colon). Stimulate all back calf points and Stomach 36. Hold pen, the point retracted, on inner and outer corners of skin near bottom of big toenail, 30 seconds each. Rub, and repeat. Do all lymphatic points five times, tapotement for one minute, venous pump fifteen times, effleurage five times, and nerve stroke. Healing visualization and affirmation.

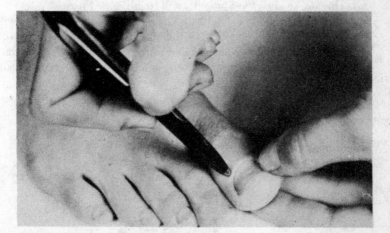

DIET

- Either fast or go on the cleansing diet.
- If you continue to eat, avoid large meals and protein. Keep the food combinations simple. Eat sprouts, especially fenugreek.

- Make a gallon of Citrus Water (page 121), and drink it freely throughout the day.

HERBS

Tea made from comfrey, fenugreek, and goldenseal is very healing. Tea made from slippery elm and thyme, with honey, sipped every few minutes, is very soothing.

ENEMA

Unless your physician has counseled otherwise, I would recommend taking an enema immediately. Make it out of goldenseal tea with one tablespoon each of lemon juice and olive oil. Optional: one tablespoon of squeezed garlic juice.

EXERCISES

- All neck rotations (see Senior Citizens), Asthma Exercise 1, and shoulder stand (see Students) will help a sore throat.
- The *Lion Pose* is an exercise which, when done regularly, will build resistance against sore throats, and strengthen the throat area. It is not to be done while having a sore throat. Sit on your heels, or in a chair with your hands on your knees. Inhale

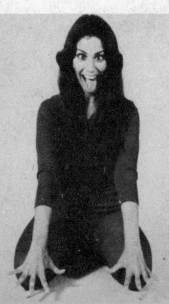

Lion Pose.

deeply. On a strong exhalation, make a long, loud noise like a lion. As you do this, tense your whole body, face, fingers, and stick your tongue out as far as it will go. The eyes stare at a point in the middle of your brows. As you do this, concentrate on the throat area, and visualize it being strengthened as blood and nutrition rush to the cells. Repeat this two more times.

Stiff Neck

REFLEXOLOGY

Rotate all toes. Work all the toe points, especially the sides of the big toe and first metatarsal. Plexus pull, and then all the ankle movements. Extension and flexion of all the toes. Hold the maximum stretch for thirty seconds each. Venous pump fifteen times. Effleurage seven times. Nerve stroke, healing visualization, and affirmation.

DIET

- Avoid pasteurized dairy products, refined foods, too many proteins at one meal, excessive eating, too many starches or acidic foods, and protein late at night.
- Drink lemon water (water with juice of one fresh lemon squeezed into it) fresh fruit and vegetable juices freely and eat fresh green salads.

EXERCISE

- Do all the rotations mentioned in the Senior Citizens program. Do these morning and night, and throughout the day whenever you have been sitting a long time.
- Avoid poor posture, sitting in poor chairs, bad shoes, tense situations, and uncomfortable suits and ties.
- Do the *Special Neck Release Exercise* for five minutes. At first it may be too tender for you to hold this long. So hold it as best you can, relax a few moments, then do it again, so that you do get at least five minutes of it.

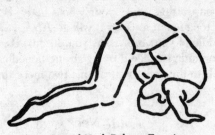

Special Neck Release Exercise.

- From a kneeling position, with the top of your head on the floor, support most of your weight with your hands, and keep your knees firmly on the floor.
- Inhale, and make sure you are relaxed. Exhale, and roll your body forward, rolling as far on the back of your head as you can, so that your neck and upper shoulder muscles feel stretched and challenged.
- Find your maximum "edge," and hold it here, while doing gentle deep breathing. Before letting go, exhale fully, and try to stretch a little further.
- This will help tight upper shoulders, neck, and tendency toward tension headaches.

It is very important to keep your neck loose and free of tension. It connects your brain and nervous system to your body. If you allow tension to remain in your neck, you are definitely operating on a deficit and on an imbalance of energy.

Tight, Weak Shoulders

REFLEXOLOGY

Rotate all the toes firmly. Do big toe release. Work on shoulder, arm, sciatic, and hip. Work on base of toes, base stretch. Nail-inching on toes, flexion and extension, plexus pull. Tapotement, venous pump, and effleurage. Nerve stroke, healing visualization, and affirmation.

DIET

- Don't overeat. Don't eat guiltily, knowing that what you're eating is bad for you. Make sure you eat about 80 per cent alkaline, 20 per cent acidic foods. Many proteins, acidic foods, and heavy greasy foods contribute to muscular aches.
- If deficient in manganese or magnesium, try taking a supplement and eating walnuts, seeds, potatoes, or corn meal.
- Avoid milk products for a few weeks.
- Take a bath with ½ cup vinegar and 2½ lbs. epsom salt. Soak for twenty minutes.

EXERCISE

- *Shoulder Drop.* Push your shoulders up toward your ears on the inhale. On a strong, hissing exhale, push them down toward the floor. Continue this up and down movement for twenty-five times.
- *Neck Rotations* (see Senior Citizens).
- *Special Neck Release Exercise* (Stiff Neck).
- *Shoulder Reach Exercise.* Exhale fully while lying on back. Inhale and lift head and shoulders up, arms and hands rising to hip level. Hold for a count of ten, relaxing the shoulders as much as possible. Exhale down. Repeat five to ten times.

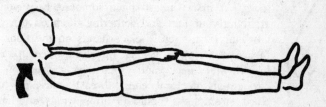

The Shoulder Reach Exercise.

- *Clasping Hands Exercise.* Try to clasp hands behind back. If not possible, hold hands at closest point on the back. Inhale and stretch the upper elbow higher up toward the ceiling. On the exhale, keep clasping hands together, as much as possible, lean forward, touching head to the floor. Hold for count of five, then inhale up. Repeat five to ten times.

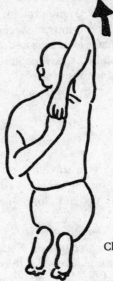

Clasping Hands Exercise.

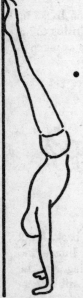

Shoulder Handstand.

- *Shoulder Handstand.* This is not nearly so hard as it looks. At first you can have someone help you by grabbing your legs and centering them on the wall. On your own, merely place hands on the floor and throw your feet up against the wall. Once up, relax breath, let neck and spine hang freely. This strengthens pectoral chest (breast) muscles, tones chest, strengthens shoulders, arms, wrists, and hands. Great for neck troubles, spinal aches anywhere. Stimulates complexion, circulation, glandular activity, and bowel activity. If you do head stands regularly you usually jam neck vertebrae together. This shoulder stand is good to do after the head stand to release the vertebrae and realign them, allowing energy to flow and shoulders to relax.

Varicose Veins

REFLEXOLOGY

Stimulate heart, glands, spine. Stimulate all toes well. Stimulate sciatic, hips, ankle movements and plexus pull. Do venous pump fifteen times at least five times a day, tapotement, effleurage fifteen times. Nerve stroke, healing visualization, and affirmation.

DIET

- Eat raw foods, whole grains, seeds, and avoid refined foods.
- Suggested supplements: 2 tsp. lecithin/day, 2 tsp. kelp/day, Vitamin C (up to 3 grams), Vitamin E (500–1000 I.U. daily), balanced B-complex or 2 T. brewer's yeast (most important are C and E).

HERBAL TEAS

Yarrow and raspberry leaf.

EXERCISE

- Slant board, head or shoulder or handstand at least twice a day.
- Don't sit for overly long periods. Get up, deep breathe, and stretch.
- Spinal rocking, long walks, and deep breathing.
- All the menstrual exercises that elevate legs and hips are good for this problem.

An Old Japanese Foot Tale

Otau was a wise, old, and wrinkled man. The whole village respected his healing abilities.

One day a foreigner came to ask him many questions and write down the healing ways of Otau.

However, all Otau would say was, "See to their feet and you have seen to their body."

"I do not understand," insisted the foreigner.

"Your understanding will never be enough," Otau chuckled. "See to their feet, and that will be enough."

Appendix of Foot Facts

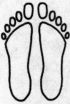 You should become acquainted with your feet. If no one else will, they'll always support you. When you sit, the base of your spine is the sacrum. When you walk, the base of your spine is your feet. Your spine and your feet are your lifeline. You are only as young as your spine is limber and your feet are healthy. Just as you check your eyes, teeth, and body at regular intervals, have your spine checked, and your feet treated.

SKELETAL STRUCTURE OF THE FOOT

The skeleton of the foot has:

    seven tarsal bones
      talus
      calcaneus
      navicular
      cuboid
      three cuneiform bones
    five metatarsal bones
      one for each digit
    fourteen phalanges
      three for four smaller digits
      two for big toe

Tibia

Fibula

Talus

Navicular

Cuneiform
Bones

Calcaneus

Cuboid

Metatarsals

Phalanges

The body weight is:

1. transmitted by the tibia to the talus . . .
2. then distributed down to the heel (calcaneus) . . .
3. and toward the metatarsals through the navicular bone.

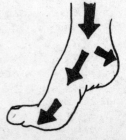

Bones of Right Foot
Dorsal (Top) View

- The metatarsals are convex in this position.

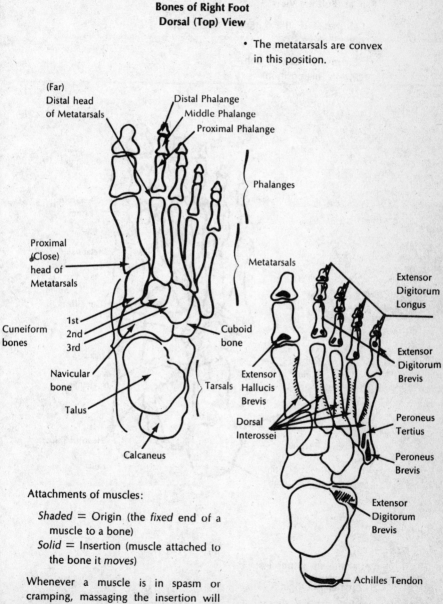

(Far)
Distal head
of Metatarsals

Distal Phalange
Middle Phalange
Proximal Phalange

Phalanges

Proximal
(Close)
head of
Metatarsals

Metatarsals

Cuneiform
bones

1st
2nd
3rd

Cuboid
bone

Navicular
bone

Tarsals

Talus

Calcaneus

Extensor
Digitorum
Longus

Extensor
Digitorum
Brevis

Extensor
Hallucis
Brevis

Peroneus
Tertius

Dorsal
Interossei

Peroneus
Brevis

Extensor
Digitorum
Brevis

Achilles Tendon

Attachments of muscles:

Shaded = Origin (the *fixed* end of a
muscle to a bone)

Solid = Insertion (muscle attached to
the bone it *moves*)

Whenever a muscle is in spasm or
cramping, massaging the insertion will
relieve this.

**Bones of Right Foot
Plantar (Bottom) View**

- Calcaneus is the largest bone (heel).

- The metatarsals are concave in this position.

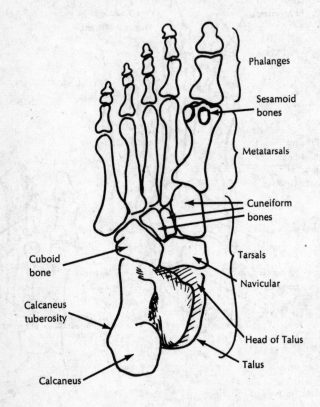

Attachments of muscles:

Shaded = Origin
Solid = Insertion

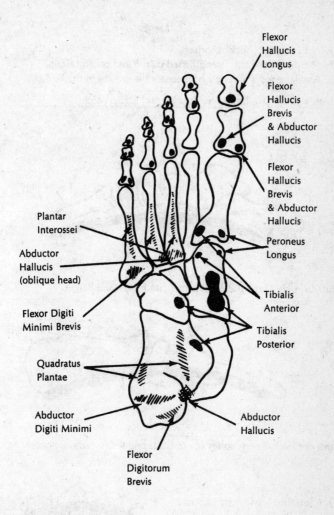

Flexor Hallucis Longus

Flexor Hallucis Brevis & Abductor Hallucis

Flexor Hallucis Brevis & Abductor Hallucis

Plantar Interossei

Abductor Hallucis (oblique head)

Peroneus Longus

Flexor Digiti Minimi Brevis

Tibialis Anterior

Tibialis Posterior

Quadratus Plantae

Abductor Digiti Minimi

Abductor Hallucis

Flexor Digitorum Brevis

Arches

1. Act as elastic shock absorbers.
2. Are stimulated and strengthened by use and rough terrain.
3. Are flattened and lengthened under the weight of the body.

Medial Arch. Five bones, the longest and highest arch

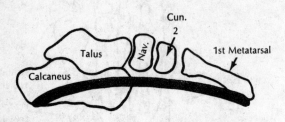

Lateral Arch. Three bones, intermediate length and height

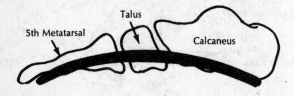

Anterior Arch. Seven bones (metatarsals and two sesamoid bones)

(The forefoot is widened 12.5 mm
under the weight of the body.)

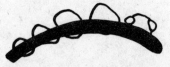

TENDONS AND MUSCLES
Tendons that Travel Around the
Outside Ankle (Lateral Ankle)

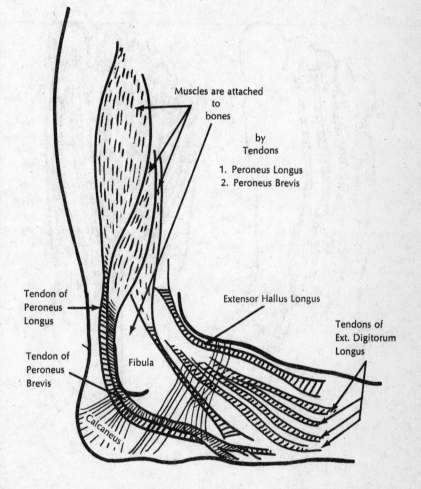

Muscles are attached
to
bones

by
Tendons

1. Peroneus Longus
2. Peroneus Brevis

Tendon of
Peroneus
Longus

Extensor Hallus Longus

Tendons of
Ext. Digitorum
Longus

Tendon of
Peroneus
Brevis

Fibula

Calcaneus

SOLE OF THE FOOT

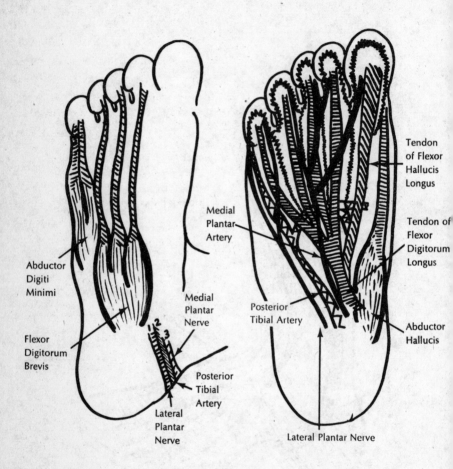

Abductor
Digiti
Minimi

Flexor
Digitorum
Brevis

Medial
Plantar
Artery

Medial
Plantar
Nerve

Posterior
Tibial
Artery

Lateral
Plantar
Nerve

Tendon
of Flexor
Hallucis
Longus

Tendon of
Flexor
Digitorum
Longus

Posterior
Tibial Artery

Abductor
Hallucis

Lateral Plantar Nerve

The Achilles Tendon is the tendon of your calf muscle attached to your heel (the gastrocnemius muscle attached to the calcaneus bone).

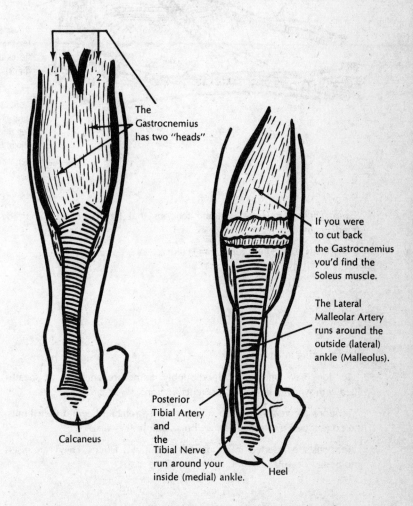

The Gastrocnemius has two "heads"

If you were to cut back the Gastrocnemius you'd find the Soleus muscle.

The Lateral Malleolar Artery runs around the outside (lateral) ankle (Malleolus).

Calcaneus

Posterior Tibial Artery and the Tibial Nerve run around your inside (medial) ankle.

Heel

* *Runners* use the gastrocnemius muscles a lot. *Walkers* use the soleus. ("You gallop with the gastrocs and stroll with the soleus . . ."—Dr. Oliver Titrud.) They both insert into the heel. Thus, for cramps, pain, or strengthening of calves, massage the insertion of Achilles Tendon onto the heel.

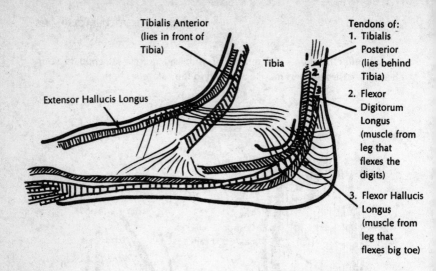

Tibialis Anterior (lies in front of Tibia)

Tibia

Tendons of:
1. Tibialis Posterior (lies behind Tibia)

Extensor Hallucis Longus

2. Flexor Digitorum Longus (muscle from leg that flexes the digits)

3. Flexor Hallucis Longus (muscle from leg that flexes big toe)

"Tom, Dick, and Harry" are the tendons that travel around the inside (medial) ankle.

T = Tibialis; D = Digitorum; H = Hallucis

It's interesting to know:

Tendons have very little blood supply. Some are enclosed in sheaths filled with synovial fluid. This prevents friction.

Tendons are very strong. So strong, that if stretched beyond their limits, the bone they are attached to may break before they do.

Tendons are inserted into bones by Sharpey's Fibers. They can insert into bone or cartilage.

LYMPHATIC SYSTEM

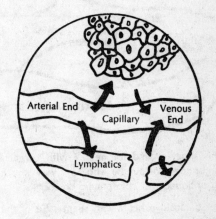

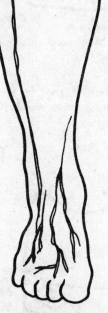

Deep Lymphatic Channels
and Nodes

All cells are bathed in tissue fluid that diffuses out of capillaries. Some draws back into capillaries. The other goes into the blind-ended, thin-walled lymph circulation. (It is equivalent to plasma without protein.)

Lymphatic vessels drain tissue spaces of poisons throughout the body, and eventually draw back into the bloodstream. As lymph moves, it ingests foreign matter or harmful bacteria (e.g. lung pollutants).

Movement of lymph toward the heart depends on:

1. Compression of lymphatics by contraction of muscles.

2. Movements of respiration.

Thus, massage and breath greatly help stimulate lymphatic cleansing, drainage.

SHOES

Good for
spines
like this

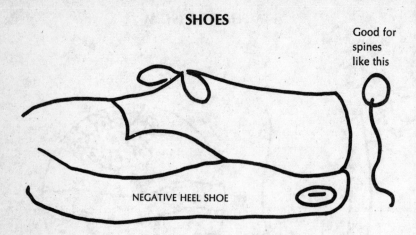

NEGATIVE HEEL SHOE

This shoe is good for people with backaches, sway backs, scoliosis. It is not good for people who have very straight lumbar spines. Check with an orthopedic or chiropractic doctor.

Flat or positive heels with slight raise of the heels are good for people with abnormally straight lumbar spines. They are not good for sway backs.

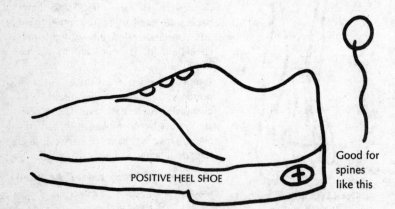

POSITIVE HEEL SHOE

Good for
spines
like this

Good shoes should have arch supports in the center that are high and firm enough, but flexible. The shoes should give support on both sides. There should be a lot of room for all the toes. They should fit snugly about the heel. Wearing sandals, gym shoes, etc., which have little support or shock absorption, is not a good habit on city streets. When in the city, have a city survival consciousness and wear appropriate shoes. However, go barefoot on natural rough terrain whenever possible.

Wearing Heels

- Toes hit against tip of shoes and
  become hyperextended, becoming claw feet (*pes cavus*).
- Metatarsal heads are thus lowered.
- Exaggerates curvature of arch.
- Shortens and tightens the calf muscles.
- This eventually leads to tightened, shortened
  spine and decrease in height.
- Can add to strain on genitals, and lower back.
- Can cause or influence tipped uterus.

- This holds true for
  men and women,
  and children, too.

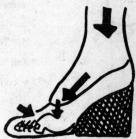

- High heels and shoes that
  are too tight pro-
  duce inversion of
  the anterior arch.

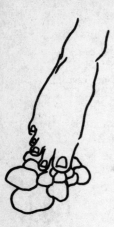

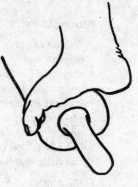

Feet are made to mold to the earth.

On uneven ground, every part of the foot is used. All the ligaments and muscles are exercised.

Flat ground and shoes with too little or too much support prevent this.

Hard, even ground and shoes take the spring and exercise out of the arches, and collapse them.

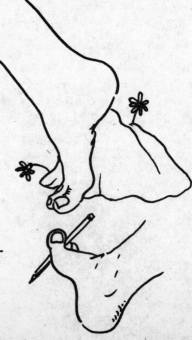

Appendix of Oils, Creams, Packs, and Footbaths

Oils

It is best to massage with oils only when the treatment is for relaxation. It is too difficult to make good therapeutic contacts with oil. When I do use a lubricant, I prefer an herbal absorbent cream.

However, since there are special situations that do call for oils, for heat, and for special packs on the area, here are some useful ones that are applied externally and may be prepared quite simply.

OIL FOR RELAXING

Mix a few drops of lavender or geranium oil with a combination of sweet almond oil, olive oil, and a small amount of mustard oil. (Castor oil will substitute for mustard.)

OIL FOR DETOXIFYING

To ¼ cup of vegetable oil (preferably sesame with some mustard oil) add the following: 3 chili pods, 15 black pepper corns, and no more than ¼ tsp. of cayenne. Simmer this mixture over a low flame for at least one hour. Before using, be sure to strain.

Massage the patient while the oil is still warm. Rub it deeply into the feet and the rest of the body if desired. Continue applying oil until the skin is saturated.

Next do tapotement for one minute, followed by General Lymphatics for one minute, then venous pump and effleurage. (This is also very good to do if the patient is on a cleansing or reducing diet.)

THERAPEUTIC OILS

The following are some oils that are fairly easy to obtain and which have interesting therapeutic value:

Camomile. This is stimulating and has the opposite effects of tea. It can be used very effectively in foot baths.

Cayenne. Cayenne oil increases circulation, tones the area to which it is applied, and detoxifies.

Cinnamon. An antiseptic.

Clove. An antiseptic.

Coriander.. Although this is a carminative, it produces a warm sensation. It is also good for getting rid of blackheads and for drying a naturally oily skin.

Garlic.. An antibiotic.

Geranium. Geranium oil revives tired skin.

Lavender. A nerve tonic and antiseptic good for general weakness and is used to reduce swelling in the limbs.

Creams

It is very difficult to make a homemade cream that is absorbent enough and still not greasy. Here is a recipe for a homemade cream you will find easy to make and which is as greaseless as "homemade possible."

A GOOD GENERAL HOMEMADE CREAM

2 T. cocoa butter (the genuine kind—not a commercial blend)
3 T. almond oil
2 T. anhydrous lanolin
2 tsp. rose water or several drops of herbal oil
½ tsp. honey

Combine the first three ingredients in a Pyrex bowl over hot water. Blend, and remove mixture from heat while still warm. When it has cooled, beat in the rose water or oil. You may even add a few drops of Vitamin E. The mixture should be kept refrigerated in a closed container.

Packs

The following packs are especially designed for application to the feet of a patient bothered by colds, the flu, or achy joints.

CASTOR OIL PACKS

Dip three layers of flannel in castor oil. Wring well. Place the flannel over the patient's feet and hold in place with rubber bands, being careful that the bands are not too tight, stopping circulation. Cover the area with plastic to protect the hot water bottle or heating pad that goes over the flannel and to keep them clean.

We should mention here that castor oil packs are especially good for sore throats.

GINGER PACKS

Grate fresh ginger root and put between two layers of flannel. The flannel should be previously dipped in hot water and wrung damp. Place the flannel over the feet and hold in place with rubber bands.

Ginger packs also combat debilitation, poor digestion, and flatulence if placed on both the abdomen and feet.

HEAT PACKS

Heat packs are recommended for muscular aches. Hot water bottles or heating pads should be placed directly over the aching joint and at the same time over the soles of the feet.

GARLIC AND ONION PACKS

Grate garlic and onion and place between two layers of moist flannel, or blend and soak three layers of flannel in the mixture. Place over soles of feet and hold in place with rubber bands. Heat from a hot water bottle or heating pad should be applied to the flannel pack unless the patient is running a fever, in which case omit the heat.

Footbaths

Start by making a strong herbal tea, using the tea that will give the therapeutic effect you are interested in, or add a few drops of the appropriate oil. An especially soothing bath is one made with strong peppermint tea, and no oils will be required. For distress from a cold, comfrey and clove tea is recommended with freshly squeezed garlic or garlic capsules added to the water.

The patient's feet should be soaked in the tea for fifteen minutes while the tea is kept comfortably warm. The feet are then brushed with a firm brush or loufa sponge under water. Keep the feet underwater and do nail stimulation and flicking on all toes.

Dry the feet and apply appropriate oil for the desired effect. The oil should be rubbed well into the skin and applied several times to saturate the skin. Follow this with venous pump, effleurage, nerve stroke, and affirmation.

A mixture of one half clove oil and one half cinnamon oil is especially nice after a footbath. Footbaths rejuvenate the entire body, especially the digestive system, the lungs, and the skin.

Appendix of Color Therapy

Color therapy has been used by healers for thousands of years. Recently, along with the surge of research on many alternative modes of healing as compared to allopathic medicine, color therapy is being rediscovered and appreciated.

The way to use color therapy to augment foot treatments is as follows:

1. Shine a colored light onto the feet as you do the treatment. Use the appropriate color for the desired effect, as described in the discussion of Colors and their Effects. Colors are produced by buying thin gel filters and taping them over the bulb of a lamp, placed four to eight feet from the patient's feet. The lamp should shine toward the feet. The gels are inexpensive, easy to use, and pure. The colors must be pure in color therapy to get the desired results. For example, pure red will have no purple hues in it.

2. Another alternative to colored light, or to be used in conjunction with colored light, is using "colored oil": Put oil in an appropriately colored jar (must be a pure color), cork, and allow to

sit in direct sunlight, outdoors, for at least twelve hours. Then use this oil on the feet, or in making homemade cream.

The authoritative book on this subject is Dr. Edwin D. Babbit's *The Principles of Light and Color*, edited by Faber Birren, University Books, New Hyde Park, New York.

By the scientific application of color, you are introducing a natural energy into the body that helps the body cleanse, repair, and heal. After all, it is no miracle, no illusion, no hype . . . you are dealing with the higher vibratory forces of nature. You are dealing with the source of all—LIGHT.

Of course, *sunlight is the great healer* and contains all the colors of the spectrum. We are discovering new healing methods, that you will soon read about, done with the prism, focusing all the colors onto people to heal them.

Do not use color therapy in the path of direct sunlight or under other harsh lights. Natural indirect lighting is fine.

You can also suggest to the patients that they wear certain colors or avoid others, to enhance their healing processes. Explain why, and they will be fascinated and receptive.

Colors and Their Effects

RED — Used to invigorate, stimulate and to give energy to the body. Good for anemia, poor blood circulation, any debilitation or coldness. Red puts a lot of iron and minerals into the blood. It is good for liver and heart problems. Do not use red on very emotional people.

PINK — Used for pelvic problems. Pink helps hip and buttock tenderness. Pink stimulates a loving feeling in the heart.

ORANGE — Used to invigorate, stimulate, and warm the emotions and the glands. Orange stimulates confidence, success, proper respiratory functioning, enhances lactation, relieves gas and sluggish digestion, helps drain and bring infections to a head. It decreases menstrual cramps. Orange is very good for people paralyzed with fears and doubts. People with thyroid trouble are helped by wearing an orange scarf around the neck.

YELLOW	Used to stimulate the nervous system and brain activity. Yellow increases receptivity for knowledge, self-confidence, appetite, enhances liver and gall bladder functions, and helps dissolve arthritic deposits.
LEMON	Used to help cleanse and loosen mucus, to activate the thymus gland in retarded children, to build bone, and to help speed up the eliminative and healing process of a cold. Lemon color relieves and soothes the body of muscular tension.
GREEN	Used for stabilizing, peaceful, and calming effects on the body and mind. Green is the neutral, master color. It is used for high blood pressure, hot flashes, menopause, and in the cases when you feel that the patient is subconsciously resisting healing. Green is said to raise the vibration of the body over that of the disease, to help overpower and heal the problem. Green stimulates the pituitary, the master gland. This is the color to use for infection in the body.
TURQUOISE	Used to deal with pain and aches, and to build up the skin for any skin affliction, including itching.
BLUE	Used to help the body deal with a feverish situation, to encourage a deep, healing sleep, and to stimulate the pineal gland.
INDIGO	Used for its sedative effects, for reducing swelling and pain caused by it, and for firming skin.
VIOLET	Used to relax and slow down the motor functioning of the body (i.e., muscles) Violet acts as an antibiotic, a builder of white corpuscles in the spleen, and depresses the appetite.
PURPLE	Used to slow the heartbeat and reduce heart pain. Purple increases venous drainage, so it is very good for stiffness, systemic congestion, and excessive menstruation.
SCARLET	Used to stimulate heartbeat and arterial action. Scarlet peps up kidneys and adrenal gland functioning.

Index

feet:
  exploration of, 22-24
  people often on, 105
  reasons for emphasis on, 6-7
  spine and, 13-14
  tender reflexes found in, 1, 4, 32-33
  washing of, 21
feet-body correlation, recent studies of,
    13-14
fertility problems, 89-90
fetus, 6, 12
fevers, child's, 97-98
final cleansing, 59
final cleansing stroke, 31
fingers, exercising for sensitivity of, 24
Fitzgerald, William H., 11
flexion and extension against resistance, 44
flexion release, 42, 49
foods (see also diet):
  acid and alkaline, 75
  classification of, 75-76
footbaths, 203-204
foot charts, study of, 5
foot facts, 187
foot reflexes, 1
  as proprioceptive nerve receptors, 16
foot reflex points (see also reflex points), 6,
    7, 12-13
  acupuncture points related to, 14
four-part visualization, 74
friction, 25

gall bladder problems, 162-164
garlic and onion packs, 203
General Lymphatics movement, 57, 62
general movements:
  in abbreviated treatment, 60
  in basic treatment, 36, 37-41
genital point, 61
Gillet, H., 13
ginger packs, 203
Gland Drink, 122
Goodheart, Dr., 16
granular deposits, 31-32
Green Drink, 142
Gunn, C. C., 16

hair, condition of, 4
hair problems, 153-154
Han, Kim Bong, 14
hands, 6, 11
  preparation of, before touching patient,
    21-22
hay fever, 177-179
head, 6
headaches, 155

healing affirmations:
  in abbreviated treatment, 62
  in basic treatment, 37, 59
healing art:
  detective role in, 4
  levels of, 3-4
  practices helpful to, 4-5
Healing Mind, The, 65
health of healer, 5
heart problems, 155-157
heart reflex, 2
heat packs, 203
heels, shoe, 4
herbs, 73
  for backache pain, 133, 134
  for common cold, 139
  for complexion problems, 140
  for constipation, 148
  for digestive problems, 142, 148
  for headaches and dizziness, 155
  for heart and circulation problems, 156
  for high blood pressure, 159
  for hypoglycemia, 161
  for low blood pressure, 165
  for menstrual problems, 167
  for pregnancy, 169
  for respiratory problems, 172
  for sinuses and allergies, 177
  for sore throats, 180
  for yeast infections, 168
high blood pressure, 158-160
Hing, M. H., 16
Hirata, Krurakichi, 12
How to Observe Toes, 13
hypoglycemia, 160-161

illnesses, childhood, 96-99
illnesses, common (see also specific ail-
    ments), 124-185
Integrated Treatment:
  as art, 8
  basic strokes in, 25-33
  basic techniques and procedures for,
    34-62
  exploration and, 22-24
  functions of, 5
  meaning of, 2-3
  mental aspect of, 8
  physical aspect of, 7-8
  preparation for, 19-22
  self-therapy in, 18
  spiritual plane of, 8
iris, 6

Japan:
  ancient healing systems in, 10
  shiatsu in, 13